Veterinary Public Health

Guest Editor

ROSALIE T. TREVEJO, DVM, PhD, MPVM

VETERINARY CLINICS OF NORTH AMERICA: SMALL ANIMAL PRACTICE

www.vetsmall.theclinics.com

March 2009 • Volume 39 • Number 2

SAUNDERS an imprint of ELSEVIER, Inc.

W.B. SAUNDERS COMPANY
A Division of Elsevier Inc.

1600 John F. Kennedy Blvd. • Suite 1800 • Philadelphia, PA 19103-2899

http://www.vetsmall.theclinics.com

VETERINARY CLINICS OF NORTH AMERICA: SMALL ANIMAL PRACTICE Volume 39, Number 2
March 2009 ISSN 0195-5616, ISBN-13: 978-1-4377-0561-4, ISBN-10: 1-4377-0561-8

Editor: John Vassallo; j.vassallo@elsevier.com
Developmental Editor: Donald Mumford

Veterinary Clinics of North America: Small Animal Practice (ISSN 0195-5616) is published bimonthly (For Pos
Office use only: volume 39 issue 2 of 6) by Elsevier Inc., 360 Park Avenue South, New York, NY 10010-1710
Months of issue are January, March, May, July, September, and November. Business and Editorial Offices
1600 John F. Kennedy Blvd., Suite 1800, Philadelphia, PA 19103-2899. Customer Service Office: 11830 West
line Industrial Drive, St. Louis, MO 63146. Periodicals postage paid at New York, NY and additional mailing of
fices. Subscription prices are $229.00 per year (domestic individuals), $366.00 per year (domestic institutions)
$114.00 per year (domestic students/residents), $303.00 per year (Canadian individuals), $450.00 per yea
(Canadian institutions), $336.00 per year (international individuals), $450.00 per year (international institutions)
and $165.00 per year (international and Canadian students/residents). To receive student/resident rate, orders
must be accompanied by name of affiliated institution, date of term, and the *signature* of program/residency
coordinator on institution letterhead. Orders will be billed at individual rate until proof of status is received
Foreign air speed delivery is included in all *Clinics* subscription prices. All prices are subject to change withou
notice. **POSTMASTER:** Send address changes to *Veterinary Clinics of North America: Small Animal Practice*
11830 Westline Industrial Drive, St. Louis, MO 63146. Customer Service (orders, claims, online, change of address)
Elsevier Periodicals Customer Service, 11830 Westline Industrial Drive, St. Louis, MO 63146. Tel: 1-800-654-2452
(U.S. and Canada). Fax: 314-523-5170. E-mail: journalscustomerservice-usa@elsevier.com (for print support)
journalsonlinesupport-usa@elsevier.com (for online support).

Reprints. For copies of 100 or more of articles in this publication, please contact the Commercial Reprints
Department, Elsevier Inc., 360 Park Avenue South, New York, NY 10010-1710. Tel.: 212-633-3812; Fax
212-462-1935; E-mail: reprints@elsevier.com.

Veterinary Clinics of North America: Small Animal Practice is also published in Japanese by Inter Zoo Publishing
Co., Ltd., Aoyama Crystal-Bldg 5F, 3-5-12 Kitaaoyama, Minato-ku, Tokyo 107-0061, Japan.

Veterinary Clinics of North America: Small Animal Practice is covered in *Current Contents/Agriculture, Biology
and Environmental Sciences, Science Citation Index, ASCA, MEDLINE/PubMed (Index Medicus), Excerpta
Medica,* and *BIOSIS.*

Printed in the United States of America.

Contributors

GUEST EDITOR

ROSALIE T. TREVEJO, DVM, PhD, MPVM
Diplomate, American College of Veterinary Preventive Medicine (Epidemiology); Adjunct Professor of Epidemiology and Public Health, College of Veterinary Medicine, Western University of Health Sciences, Pomona, California

AUTHORS

EMILY BEELER, DVM
Zoonosis Veterinarian, Los Angeles County Department of Public Health, Veterinary Public Health and Rabies Control Program, Downey; Adjunct Professor, College of Veterinary Medicine, Western University of Health Sciences, Pomona, California

JEFF B. BENDER, DVM, MS
Diplomate, American College of Veterinary Preventive Medicine; Associate Professor, Veterinary Public Health, University of Minnesota, St. Paul, Minnesota

GUNDULA DUNNE, DVM, MPVM
Diplomate; American College of Veterinary Preventive Medicine; Veterinary Medical Officer, County of San Diego, Department of Agriculture, Weights, and Measures, Office of the County Veterinarian, Animal Disease Diagnostic Laboratory, San Diego, California

KAREN EHNERT, DVM, MPVM
Diplomate, American College of Veterinary Preventive Medicine; Senior Veterinarian, Los Angeles County Department of Public Health, Veterinary Public Health & Rabies Control, Downey; Adjunct Associate Professor, College of Veterinary Medicine, Western University of Health Sciences, Pomona, California

HELEN T. ENGELKE, BVSc, MPVM, MRCVS
Assistant Professor of Veterinary Public Health, College of Veterinary Medicine, Western University of Health Sciences, Pomona, California

ERIKA FRIEDMANN, PhD
Professor, University of Maryland School of Nursing, Baltimore, Maryland

CURTIS L. FRITZ, DVM, MPVM, PhD
Diplomate, American College of Veterinary Preventive Medicine (Epidemiology); Research Scientist IV (Epidemiology/Biostatistics), Division of Communicable Disease Control, California Department of Public Health, Sacramento, California

G. GALE GALLAND, DVM, MS
Captain, United States Public Health Services, Centers for Disease Control and Prevention, Division of Global Migration and Quarantine, Atlanta, Georgia

iv Contributors

NIKOS GURFIELD, DVM
Diplomate, American College of Veterinary Pathology; County Veterinarian, County of San Diego, Department of Agriculture, Weights, and Measures, Office of the County Veterinarian, Animal Disease Diagnostic Laboratory, San Diego, California

ELIZABETH LUND, DVM, MPH, PhD
Senior Director of Research, Banfield, The Pet Hospital, Portland, Oregon

GEORGE E. MOORE, DVM, MS, PhD
Associate Professor, Department of Comparative Pathobiology, School of Veterinary Medicine, Purdue University, West Lafayette, Indiana

PEGGY L. SCHMIDT, DVM, MS
Diplomate, American College of Veterinary Preventative Medicine; Associate Professor of Population Health and Epidemiology, and Director of Year 4 Curriculum, College of Veterinary Medicine, Western University of Health Sciences, Pomona, California; Adjunct Assistant Professor, School of Public Health, University of Minnesota, Minneapolis, Minnesota

HEESOOK SON, MPH, RN
PhD Student, University of Maryland School of Nursing, Baltimore, Maryland

ROSALIE T. TREVEJO, DVM, PhD, MPVM
Diplomate, American College of Veterinary Preventive Medicine (Epidemiology); Adjunct Professor of Epidemiology and Public Health, College of Veterinary Medicine, Western University of Health Sciences, Pomona, California

JAMIE K. UMBER, DVM
Post Doctoral Associate, Veterinary Population Medicine, University of Minnesota, St. Paul, Minnesota

VICTORIA L. VOITH, DVM, PhD
Diplomate, American College of Veterinary Behaviorists; Professor of Animal Behavior, College of Veterinary Medicine, Western University of Health Sciences, Pomona, California

Contents

All veterinarians, regardless of their formal job description, serve the public good and contribute to public health. The public health activities veterinarians engage in most frequently in clinical practice are in the areas of disease detection, reporting, and prevention. This article provides a brief overview of the basic functions of public health, while emphasizing the public health roles that veterinary clinicians play in their day-to-day practice of veterinary medicine and how they might extend their interest and involvement in this field. The multidisciplinary nature of the field of public health and the benefits of collaboration with other health care and public health professionals are also discussed.

Disease surveillance and reporting is a necessary and integral part of public health practice. Surveillance systems have been developed over many years for both human medicine and veterinary medicine. However, these systems are not usually interconnected. Today, with the benefits of advanced information technology, the development and integration of existing and new resources in companion-animal practice should be focused on "one medicine—one health" for the betterment and health of all species. This means more sharing of surveillance data, greater cooperation among organizations involved in surveillance, and further integration of human and animal surveillance activities.

Animal sentinel surveillance is a key component of public health risk assessment. While many species serve as animal sentinels, companion animals have an especially valuable role as sentinels because of their unique place in people's lives, with exposure to similar household and recreational risk factors as those for the people who own them. Dogs and cats can help in early identification of food contamination, infectious disease transmission, environmental contamination, and even bioterrorism or chemical terrorism events. Early detection, leading to early intervention, can minimize the impact of these adverse events on both animal and human health.

Influenza has been long absent from the list of infectious diseases considered as possibilities in dogs and cats. With the discovery that avian influenza H5N1 can infect cats and dogs, and the appearance of canine influenza H3N8, small animal veterinarians have an important role to play in detection of influenza virus strains that may become zoonotic. Small animal veterinarians must educate staff and clients about influenza to improve understanding as to when and where influenza infection is possible, and to avert unreasonable fears.

Ticks are capable of transmitting numerous pathogens to both humans and their pets. The risks of tick-borne disease risks vary geographically and are determined by the climate, environment, the presence of rodents and other mammal reservoirs, and the species of ticks parasitizing wild and domestic animals. Zoonoses such as Lyme borreliosis, tularemia, and tick-borne rickettsioses can emerge in previously nonendemic areas when circumstances favorable to their maintenance and transmission arise. Tick-borne zoonosis can be prevented by implementation and adoption of an integrated program to reduce the likelihood of tick bites on pets and their owners.

Antimicrobial resistance is a growing problem and is a significant public health issue. An increasing number of organisms are developing resistance to many of the antimicrobial agents available for treatment of infections in both humans and animals. These resistant organisms often result in greater disease severity, longer hospitalization, and increased care and treatment costs. This article reviews the current situation of antimicrobial resistance in companion small animals and highlights how important it is for veterinarians to recognize the significance of antimicrobial resistance and to commit to the judicious use of antimicrobial agents.

Changes in the global trade market have led to a thriving international pet trade in exotic animals, birds, and puppies. The flood of animals crossing the United States' borders satisfies the public demand for these pets but is not without risk. Imported pets may be infected with diseases that put animals or the public at risk. Numerous agencies work together to reduce the risk of animal disease introduction, but regulations may need to be modified to ensure compliance. With more than 280,000 dogs and 183,000 wildlife shipments being imported into the United States each year, veterinarians must remain vigilant so they can recognize potential threats quickly.

The San Diego County Animal Disease Diagnostic Laboratory (ADDL) is unique in its emphasis on protecting both human and animal health in San Diego County, and its use of interagency and community collaboration to create strong, effective public health programs. This article describes the ADDL core programs of avian and vector-borne disease surveillance, rabies testing, and animal abuse investigations and uses selected case studies to illustrate the need for a local veterinary diagnostic laboratory to safeguard the health of humans and animals. The ADDL serves as a role model for other local communities to develop vital public health partnerships to ensure a healthier community.

THE CLINICS ARE NOW AVAILABLE ONLINE!

Access your subscription at:
www.theclinics.com

Preface

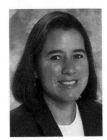

Rosalie T. Trevejo, DVM, PhD, MPVM
Guest Editor

As a veterinarian working in public health settings for much of my career, I have often found it challenging to explain what I do for a living to friends and family members, who are mystified as to why it does not involve providing direct medical care to dogs and cats. Events like the bioterrorist attacks of October 2001, during which purified *Bacillus anthracis* spores reached their victims through the U.S. mail, have obviated the need for further explanation. The popular media has brought the drama of public health into the living rooms of every one of us, such that we all now recognize its importance.

In terms of health, we are increasingly becoming "one world," with a level of inter-connectedness to our global neighbors that effectively puts us only a plane ride or cargo shipment away from one another. The level of international trade in goods and animals has made it easier for each of us to be impacted directly by events and circumstances that originate on the other side of the world. Diseases such as severe acute respiratory syndrome, monkeypox, and influenza have traveled the globe to produce human outbreaks. Given trends in pet ownership, habitat change, and global trade, we cannot ignore the reality that the health of humans, animals, and ecosystems are inextricably linked. While the concept of One Health is far from new, circumstances like the threat of bioterrorism and pandemic influenza have served to galvanize an unprecedented level of support from a wide array of health professionals to this movement. To be truly effective, this has to be a grassroots movement with participation by all veterinarians, regardless of whether they practice small animal medicine, conduct biomedical research, or coordinate mass vaccination campaigns at the international level.

This issue is not intended to be an exhaustive account of every major public health issue. Rather, the first article starts by providing a brief overview of the field and how veterinarians in clinical practice play a vital role in public health. The next two articles provide a description of the structure and function of disease detection and surveillance, which is the backbone of public health that provides the data on which sound public health practices are based. The next three articles focus on selected emerging disease topics: influenza, tick-borne diseases, and antibiotic resistance. These are followed by two articles that delve into the human-animal bond, its impact on human health, and how veterinarians play an essential role in addressing some of the animal

Vet Clin Small Anim 39 (2009) xi–xii
doi:10.1016/j.cvsm.2008.10.017
0195-5616/08/$ – see front matter

problems that have an impact on public health, such as animal bites and destructive behaviors. The article on emergency management for disasters provides an overview of existing infrastructure and describes how veterinarians can lend their expertise to this essential function. The article on border health provides the basis for understanding the impact international animal trafficking has on public health. The final article provides a case study of how San Diego County, California has capitalized on interdisciplinary collaboration to further the goals of public health and better serve all members of their community.

The major point I want the reader to take away from this issue is that no profession or government agency can effectively address all of a community's public health concerns alone. While veterinarians have long played a role in public health, the days of public health as a small subspecialty of veterinary medicine are over. The public health needs of our local communities, nation, and the world are too great; every veterinarian must play a public health role, whether it is their predominant job description or it is intermingled with their daily activities in a clinical setting. If anything, it is my hope that the readers of this issue will recognize the importance of their roles in this dynamic and be motivated to expand on that role by connecting with their local public health agencies and health care professionals outside of veterinary medicine. Methods could be simply to make an introduction, get involved in disaster planning or response efforts, deliver educational materials, or establish a mutually beneficial partnership to share diagnostic or laboratory expertise and resources. In doing so, veterinarians also play an educational role by increasing the community's awareness of our unique expertise in areas like comparative medicine and population health. With continued outreach and community involvement, the full potential of veterinary contributions to public health can be realized.

Rosalie T. Trevejo, DVM, PhD, MPVM
College of Veterinary Medicine
Western University of Health Sciences
309 East 2nd Street
Pomona, CA 91766-1854, USA

E-mail address:
rttrevejo@yahoo.com (R.T. Trevejo)

Public Health for the Twenty-First Century: What Role Do Veterinarians in Clinical Practice Play?

Rosalie T. Trevejo, DVM, PhD, MPVM

KEYWORDS

• Public health • One health • Disease reporting
• Disease surveillance • Health education

A number of events around the turn of the twentieth century heightened our society's awareness of zoonotic diseases, the role of animals in society, and how the unique expertise of veterinarians in such areas as population health and comparative medicine help address public health problems. In 1999, following observation of increased morbidity and mortality among birds, horses, and humans, West Nile virus was first detected in the Western Hemisphere.[1,2] In 2001, dried and purified *Bacillis anthracis* spores sent through the United States mail resulted in 22 persons becoming ill, leading to 5 fatalities, and over 10,000 persons being recommended antimicrobial prophylaxis.[3] When Hurricanes Katrina and Rita struck the Gulf Coast region in 2005, reports about residents who refused to abandon their pets during an evacuation and the plight of animals left behind made glaringly obvious the adverse consequences of failure to include animals in disaster plans.[4] These events have expanded the perceptions of many in government agencies and the general public regarding the roles that veterinarians play in maintaining public health and during public health crises.

Within the realm of veterinary medicine, public health is traditionally viewed as the investigation, prevention, and control of exclusively zoonotic diseases, such as rabies, psittacosis, and brucellosis. However, in reality, veterinarians lend their expertise to address a multitude of community health concerns, including emerging diseases, disaster preparedness and response, occupational health, bioterrorism, and environmental health. Most public health veterinarians work in settings that focus primarily on human-centered population health and food safety, such as in the uniformed services (eg, US Army, Air Force, and Public Health Service) and in government agencies (eg, Centers for Disease Control and Prevention, US Department of Agriculture, Food and

College of Veterinary Medicine, Western University of Health Sciences, 309 East 2nd Street, Pomona, CA 91766-1854, USA
E-mail address: rttrevejo@yahoo.com

Vet Clin Small Anim 39 (2009) 215–224
doi:10.1016/j.cvsm.2008.10.008
0195-5616/08/$ – see front matter © 2009 Elsevier Inc. All rights reserved.

Drug Administration, and state and local public health departments).[5] Less than 4% of veterinarians in the United States hold positions in the uniformed services or federal, state, or local government agencies.[6] However, all veterinarians, regardless of their formal job description, serve the public good and contribute to public health. The Veterinarian's Oath states that "the promotion of public health" is a primary function of the practice of veterinary medicine,[7] regardless of setting or specialty (**Box 1**).

To be effective, public health officials do not operate in a vacuum, but rather in concert with a number of community, governmental, commercial, and private entities and partners, including veterinary practitioners. This article provides a brief overview of the basic functions of public health, while emphasizing the roles that clinicians play in public health in their day-to-day practice of veterinary medicine, and how they might extend their interest and involvement in this field.

When discussing public health, it is useful to consider its definition. Charles Winslow, a public health visionary in the early twentieth century who had a great influence on the development of public health services in the United States, defined it as "the science and art of preventing disease, prolonging life, and promoting health and efficiency through organized community effort."[8] The World Health Organization defines veterinary public health as "the sum of all contributions to the physical, mental, and social well-being of humans, through an understanding and application of veterinary science."[9] This article uses the broader term *public health* rather than *veterinary public health* to reflect the multidisciplinary nature of the field, which relies on collaboration among many professions, including physicians, veterinarians, nurses, microbiologists, pathologists, and ecologists. A joint publication by the Board on Health Promotion and Disease Prevention and the Institute of Medicine promotes a collaborative approach to addressing public health challenges through cultivation of a "well-educated interdisciplinary cadre of public health professionals who focus on population health and understand the multiple determinants that affect health."[10] Further emblematic of the convergence of animal, human, and ecosystem health is the recent collaboration of the American Veterinary Medical Association and American Medical Association on the One Health Initiative to address "areas of mutual medical interest, such as pandemic influenza, bioterrorism risks, and biomedical research."[11] The recently released report of the American Veterinary Medical Association One Health Initiative Task Force is a call to action for individuals and professions to create partnerships to improve health worldwide.[12] It is anticipated that such developments will further expand and enhance the participation of veterinarians in the development and maintenance of healthy communities.

The practice of public health can be divided into several integrated functions, including (1) disease detection and reporting, (2) disease surveillance, (3) response, (4) health education and disease prevention, (5) program evaluation, and (6) research. The activities of veterinarians in clinical practice most frequently address the areas of

---

Box 1
Veterinarian's Oath

Being admitted to the profession of veterinary medicine, I solemnly swear to use my scientific knowledge and skills for the benefit of society through the protection of animal health, the relief of animal suffering, the conservation of livestock resources, the promotion of public health, and the advancement of medical knowledge.

I will practice my profession conscientiously, with dignity, and in keeping with the principles of veterinary medical ethics.

I accept as a lifelong obligation the continual improvement of my professional knowledge and competence.

disease detection, reporting, and prevention, though veterinarians may be involved in any of these functions to varying degrees. Each of these functions is discussed more in depth in the following sections, with the emphasis on those most directly related to clinical practice.

DISEASE DETECTION AND REPORTING

Clinicians in the front line to evaluate patients daily are in the best position to detect unusual diseases or potential disease outbreaks. Many diseases that affect animals also have public health implications because they are zoonotic, provide an early warning system for risk of human infection (ie, sentinels), or are economically important. **Table 1** lists some examples of diseases that a veterinarian working in a small-animal clinic may encounter.

Unfortunately, the agencies and processes by which reportable diseases are designated and reported are mostly independent for human and animal conditions. The Council of State and Territorial Epidemiologists composes a list of human diseases that state public health agencies report through the National Notifiable Diseases Surveillance System to the Centers for Disease Control and Prevention. As of 2008, the only animal condition reportable under this framework is rabies.[13] A separate list of nationally reportable animal conditions under the US Department of Agriculture's National Animal Health Reporting System[14] consists mainly of those diseases considered of economic concern to the livestock industry, such as foreign animal diseases. In addition to the nationally reportable diseases, each state public health and agricultural agency can require that health care providers report to their local or state agencies additional human and animal conditions of regional concern.

Because states and localities can vary about which human and animal diseases must be reported, veterinarians must maintain open lines of communication with local public health officials to find out what the local disease-reporting requirements are. A 2004 survey of over 4000 randomly selected veterinarians from New Hampshire, New Jersey, New York, and Pennsylvania found that 28% did not know if their community had a local public health agency.[15] Although veterinarians may often be required to report reportable zoonotic diseases to state agencies, rather than to local health agencies, communication with local public health officials facilitates a more coordinated and timely response to such events as disease outbreaks.[15] In addition, veterinarians may have a patient with signs that are consistent with those of a reportable condition, but no confirmation of the etiology, in which case local public health officials may be able to provide timely consultation on diseases of public health importance and access to diagnostic resources.

The growing recognition of animals as sentinels of public health events and of the frequent overlap between the health of humans and animals sharing the same environment has led to a greater appreciation of the value of having an integrated approach to disease detection and reporting. An integrated, streamlined approach that reduces the number of agencies and officials involved could facilitate a higher level of disease reporting, ensure more timely response, and foster closer collaboration between veterinarians and public health agencies. Given the potential for introduction of emerging pathogens (most of which are zoonotic)[16,17] and threat of bioterrorism,[18,19] veterinarians are a vital part of the disease-reporting network.

DISEASE SURVEILLANCE

The rote accumulation of disease reports is a fruitless exercise if those data are not used to motivate public health action. Surveillance is defined as the ongoing,

Table 1
Examples of diseases of public health significance that can affect small animals

Disease	Public Health Relevance	Species Affected	Mode of Transmission	Example
Plague (*Yesinia pestis*)	Zoonotic; animal sentinel	Mainly rodents and rabbits; also cats, dogs (rare) and humans[18]	Mainly bite of infected flea; also respiratory aerosol	23 cases of cat-associated human plague in United States from 1977 to 1998[37]
Rabies (genus *Lyssavirus*)	Zoonotic; animal sentinel; economic (cost of postexposure prophylaxis)	In United States, mostly raccoons, insectivorous bats, and skunks[38]	Mainly bite or scratch from infected animal	665 persons received postexposure prophylaxis following exposure to rabid kitten[39]
Rocky Mountain spotted fever (*Rickettsia rickettsii*)	Zoonotic; animal sentinel	Humans, dogs, rodents[40]	Bite of infected tick	Fatal human case preceded by death of owner's two dogs[41]
Salmonella spp	Zoonotic; economic	Poultry, swine, cattle, horses, dogs, cats, wild mammals and birds, reptiles, amphibians, crustaceans[42]	Food-borne and fecal-oral	Outbreaks of *S typhimurium* in 3 companion-animal clinics and 1 animal shelter; culture confirmation in 18 human and 36 animals[43]
Screwworm (*Cochliomyia hominivorax*)	Zoonotic; animal sentinel; economic	Mostly domestic livestock; rare in humans[44]	Eggs deposited directly in host tissue by female fly	Larvae detected in dog imported from Panama, preempting reintroduction into United States livestock[45]

systematic collection, analysis, and interpretation of outcome data.[20] This function is performed by public agencies, which often disseminate the data to such consumers as the health care workers who supply the disease reports, public health officials, researchers, and the scientific and popular media. Consumers can use the data to gain a better understanding of disease prevalence and trends in the community; to determine the need for new public health programs; to serve as the basis for epidemiologic studies and evaluation of public health programs; and to inform the public of preventive measures they can take to reduce their risk of illness.

The existence of disparate tracks for disease-reporting systems for humans and animals, as discussed above, often limits the quality and usefulness of these surveillance data to the community. Moreover, neither system efficiently captures data from the small-animal clinic setting. For any given disease, there may be human data but no animal data, or vice versa Or, if data exist for both animals and humans, they may have been collected under different criteria, in different data formats, or with varying degrees of completeness, making direct comparisons impossible. As a result, coordination among public agencies is hindered. An example of the kind of coordinated surveillance that can be achieved is the surveillance system developed in response to the importation of West Nile virus in 1999. In this multipronged system, data from humans (clinical cases and asymptomatic blood donors), animals (horses, wild birds, sentinel chickens), and vectors (mosquitoes) are collected by numerous state and local agencies using mutually agreed upon surveillance guidelines, then submitted to the Centers for Disease Control and Prevention for collation.[21] The existence of integrated surveillance data for West Nile virus further facilitates coordination among stakeholders by allowing consideration of animal data as a predictor of human cases. For instance, increases in crow mortality due to West Nile virus have been shown to be predictive of human cases.[22] Other factors that serve as a measure of arboviral transmission risk, and are consequently used by local agencies to direct their mosquito adulticiding and larviciding efforts, include environmental or climactic conditions, abundance of mosquito vectors, virus infection rate of mosquito vectors, sentinel chicken serovoncersions, and human infections.[23] Such integrated surveillance provides one potential model for the development of a surveillance system to facilitate standardized reporting of all reportable conditions from both animals and humans. Unfortunately such integrated surveillance is currently the exception rather than the rule.

RESPONSE

Local, state, and federal public health and agricultural agencies respond to a variety of community concerns, ranging from the seemingly common, such as routine inspection of sanitation and food-handling practices at restaurants, to the catastrophic, such as dealing with the aftermath of a large-scale earthquake. These agencies are assigned the task of providing a coordinated response to such events as disease outbreaks and natural and man-made disasters (ie, bioterrorism and agroterrorism). Many public health officials, including veterinarians, focus primarily on preparedness and response for natural and manmade disasters. In addition, veterinarians participate in the many volunteer and nonprofit animal response groups that work closely with government agencies to provide assistance with disaster response. For instance, veterinarians, animal health technicians, pharmacists, epidemiologists, safety officers, logisticians, communications specialists, and other support personnel can volunteer for the National Veterinary Response Team to assist with animal care, animal-related issues, and public health during disasters.[24,25] Veterinarians in the private practice sector can also participate in disaster relief efforts through state and local animal-response teams. As the majority of veterinarians are employed in small-animal practice,[6] having these veterinarians available to serve in a surge capacity as regulatory veterinarians or disaster responders during times of public health crises could constitute an invaluable resource to our nation's response capabilities.[26] Small-animal veterinarians could be readied to mobilize in such capacities through government-administered accreditation processes, similar to the US Department of Agriculture's voluntary National Veterinary Accreditation Program.[26] Given the potential scale of some disasters and the constant threat of bioterrorism, agroterrorism, and accidental introduction of emerging and foreign animal diseases, there is a real need for veterinarians, with their expertise in such areas as population health, comparative medicine, zoonotic diseases, and emergency medicine, to get involved in planning and response efforts.

EDUCATION AND DISEASE PREVENTION

Veterinarians are an important source of information for their clients on such public health topics as zoonotic diseases, dog-bite prevention, and disaster planning for pets. A survey of pet owners found that they acquired pet information more frequently from their veterinarian than from friends or family or from the World Wide Web, and they reported more confidence in information received from veterinarians than from other sources.[27] As such, veterinarians are in a position to proactively educate their clients as well as correct erroneous information they may receive from other sources, including other health care providers or the popular media.

There are multiple opportunities to educate clients within the small-animal hospital environment. The most direct approach is to engage the client in a discussion of preventative measures for zoonotic and chronic diseases, such as control of intestinal and ectoparasites and the importance of regular exercise, good nutrition, and vaccinations. Data from Banfield, the Pet Hospital, for 2007 show that 3.5% of canine patients and 5% of feline patients had a diagnosis of a zoonotic disease, such as roundworm, hookworm, or tapeworm infection, all of which can be prevented by deworming, use of flea control products, and good hygiene practices.[28] Such a discussion of preventive health measures could be incorporated into routine wellness visits, particularly those for puppies and kittens. This is also golden opportunity for the veterinarian to highlight the inextricable link between human and animal health by illustrating our common risk for many conditions, including tick-borne diseases, enteric pathogens, and obesity. Educational brochures, posters, and videos in waiting areas and examination rooms can serve as excellent sources of additional information for clients and help them focus on specific topics or questions of interest to discuss with the veterinarian, thereby optimizing the use of the time spent during the office visit. There are many good resources available on the Internet, including those offered by the American Veterinary Medical Association,[29] the Center for Food Security and Public Health,[30] and the Centers for Disease Control and Prevention,[31] to which veterinarians can refer as well as direct their clients.

Another area where veterinarians can have a positive impact is through community involvement and outreach.[32] For instance, veterinarians can share educational resources or deliver a presentation to members of organizations, such as schools, children's clubs (eg, Boy Scouts), church groups, service organizations (eg, Rotary Club), and senior citizen groups. In addition, the small-animal veterinarian should reach out to organizations and associations of other health care providers, such as physicians, nurses, pharmacists, and dentists, to provide information on such topics as zoonotic and emerging diseases, animals as sentinels, or the epidemiology of animal-bite injuries. Such outreach efforts also serve to establish a dialog with other partners in administering to the health of the community. Veterinarians should take every opportunity to raise awareness among health providers, health care organizations, and the public at large of specific health topics and of the diverse contributions of veterinarians to the human-animal bond, food safety, zoonotic disease prevention, and environmental health.[32]

Public health agencies and nonprofit groups often undertake large-scale disease education and prevention campaigns directed at the public. These campaigns disseminate information through various forums, including public service announcements, media interviews, print media, and posters. Some recent topics have included mosquito avoidance to reduce the risk of West Nile virus[33] and safe food-handling practices to reduce the incidence of food-borne illness.[34] Veterinarians in public agencies are often a central part of such campaigns.

PROGRAM EVALUATION

When a disease education or prevention campaign is implemented, typically by a government or nonprofit agency, the primary outcome of interest is the impact of the program (ie, did it produce the desired effect on the target population?). This measurement process can be viewed as a systematic way to improve and account for public health actions.[35] Without such feedback, it is not possible to objectively gauge how effectively program money and resources are being spent. Such information can be gathered using a variety of research techniques, including administration of surveys on attitudes, knowledge, and behaviors before and following the campaign or evaluation of surveillance data to determine if rates for the condition or behavior of interest changed following the campaign. For example, an oral rabies vaccination campaign targeting coyotes and gray foxes in Texas was evaluated by comparison of prevalence of protective immunity in targeted species before and after the vaccination campaign.[36]

OTHER RESEARCH

Other forms of public health research can encompass a wide range of activities, including those directed toward learning more about the development of antibiotic resistance and the transmission, epidemiology, treatment, and prevention of infectious diseases. This process of discovery also encompasses noninfectious conditions, such as mental health, cancer, heart disease, and injury. Veterinarians are a vital part of this research landscape, whether at academic institutions, government or nonprofit agencies, or clinical practices. For instance, veterinarians in clinical practice are involved in research efforts in various ways. They publish case reports that stimulate further studies, assist researchers with the identification of study populations, oversee clinical trials, and partner with researchers to observe and collect outcome data. The ultimate goal of public health research is the improvement in the health of humans and animals, and protection of the environment.

SUMMARY

The small-animal clinician plays many roles in protecting the health of the community. Rather than practicing in a vacuum, clinical veterinarians are in an ideal position to detect activity, such as disease outbreaks or emerging diseases, that is highly relevant to others in the community. In addition, veterinarians are a valuable resource for educating their clients, other health professionals, and the general public on many topics, including zoonotic diseases, bioterrorism, disaster preparedness for pets, and dog-bite prevention. Clinicians and local health agencies both stand to benefit from a close working relationship that is open to collaboration. Although the majority of local health departments do not have a veterinarian on staff, other officials, such as the health officer, public health nurses, and microbiologists, can all be valuable resources to veterinarians who wish to consult on cases of suspected public health significance or to submit specimens for diagnostic testing. Local health officials in turn benefit from having a veterinary resource to consult with as well as additional sets of eyes and ears in the community to alert them to events of potential public health significance. Through coordination and open lines of communication with other health care providers, public health agency officials, and the general public, the full contributions of veterinarians to the community can be realized.

REFERENCES

1. CDC. Outbreak of West Nile-like viral encephalitis—New York, 1999. MMWR Morb Mortal Wkly Rep 1999;48(38):845–9.
2. Trock SC, Meade BJ, Glaser AL, et al. West Nile virus outbreak among horses in New York state, 1999 and 2000. Emerging Infect Dis 2001;7(4):745–7.
3. Jernigan DB, Raghunathan PL, Bell BP, et al. Investigation of bioterrorism-related anthrax, United States, 2001: epidemiologic findings. Emerg Infect Dis 2002; 8(10):1019–28.
4. Nolen RS. Hurricane Katrina. Katrina's other victims. J Am Vet Med Assoc 2005; 227(8):1215–6.
5. Johnston WB. National Association of State Public Health Veterinarians: about state public health veterinarians. Available at: http://www.nasphv.org/about PHVs.html. Accessed May 27, 2008.
6. American Veterinary Medical Association. AVMA Report on Veterinary Compensation. Schaumburg (IL). 2007 edition. 1997.
7. AVMA. AVMA news: Veterinarian's Oath reaffirmed. Available at: http://www.avma. org/onlnews/javma/jun04/040601t.asp. Accessed May 29, 2008.
8. Winslow C-EA. The untilled fields of public health. Science 1920;51:23–33.
9. Who. WHO: zoonoses and veterinary public health. Available at: http://www. who.int/zoonoses/vph_intro/en/. Accessed May 28, 2008.
10. HPDP IOM. The future of public health education. In: Gebbie K, Rosenstock L, Hernandez LM, editors. Who will keep the public healthy? Educating public health professionals for the 21st century. Washington, DC: National Academy Press; 2003. p. 61–107.
11. AVMA. Press release: AMA joins AVMA "One Health" initiative to strengthen medicine by working together. Available at: http://www.avma.org/press/releases/ 070626_one_health_initiative.asp. Accessed May 28, 2008.
12. King LJ, Anderson LR, Blackmore CG, et al. Executive summary of the AVMA One Health Initiative Task Force report. J Am Vet Med Assoc 2008;233(2):259–61.
13. CDC. Nationally notifiable infectious diseases, United States. Available at: http://www. cdc.gov/ncphi/disss/nndss/phs/infdis2008.htm. 2008. Accessed May 31, 2008.
14. USDA. Animal health monitoring and surveillance: status of reportable diseases in the United States. Available at: http://www.aphis.usda.gov/vs/nahss/disease_ status.htm. Accessed May 31, 2008.
15. Kahn LH. Confronting zoonoses, linking human and veterinary medicine. Emerging Infect Dis 2006;12(4):556–61.

16. Reeves WC. The threat of exotic arbovirus introductions into California. Paper presented at the proceedings and papers of the sixty-eighth annual conference of the California Mosquito and Vector Control Association; January 2000. p. 9–10.
17. IOM. Emerging infections: microbial threats to health in the United States. Washington, DC: Institute of Medicine of the National Academy of Sciences; 1992.
18. Davis RG. The ABCs of bioterrorism for veterinarians, focusing on category A agents. J Am Vet Med Assoc 2004;224(7):1084–95.
19. Davis RG. The ABCs of bioterrorism for veterinarians, focusing on category B and C agents. J Am Vet Med Assoc 2004;224(7):1096–104.
20. Thacker SB, Berkelman RL. Public health surveillance in the United States. Epidemiol Rev 1988;10:164–90.
21. CDC. Epidemic/epizootic West Nile virus in the United States: guidelines for surveillance, prevention, and control. Available at: http://www.cdc.gov/ncidod/dvbid/westnile/resources/wnv-guidelines-aug-2003.pdf. Accessed August 3, 2008.
22. Johnson GD, Eidson M, Schmit K, et al. Geographic prediction of human onset of West Nile virus using dead crow clusters: an evaluation of year 2002 data in New York state. Am J Epidemiol 2006;163(2):171–80.
23. CDPH. California mosquito-borne virus surveillance and response plan. Available at: http://www.westnile.ca.gov/resources.php. Accessed August 3, 2008.
24. AVMA. Animal health: veterinary medical assistance teams. Available at: http://www.avma.org/disaster/vmat/default.asp. Accessed June 3, 2008.
25. DHHS. National Veterinary Response Team. Available at: http://www.hhs.gov/aspr/opeo/ndms/teams/vmat.html. Accessed June 3, 2008.
26. Wohl JS, Nusbaum KE. Public health roles for small animal practitioners. J Am Vet Med Assoc 2007;230(4):494–500.
27. Kogan LR, Goldwaser G, Stewart SM, et al. Sources and frequency of use of pet health information and level of confidence in information accuracy, as reported by owners visiting small animal veterinary practices. J Am Vet Med Assoc 2008;232(10):1536–42.
28. E. Lund Preventing zoonotic diseases. Available at: http://veterinarybusiness.dvm360.com/vetec/Veterinary+business/Preventing-zoonotic-diseases/ArticleStandard/Article/detail/535254.
29. AVMA. American Veterinary Medical Association. Available at: http://www.avma.org/. Accessed July 17, 2008.
30. CFSPH. The Center for Food Security and Public Health. Available at: http://www.cfsph.iastate.edu/. Accessed July 17, 2008.
31. CDC. Centers for Disease Control and Prevention. Available at: http://www.cdc.gov/. Accessed July 17, 2008.
32. Hendrix CM, McClelland CL, Thompson I. A punch list for changing veterinary medicine's public image in the 21st century. J Am Vet Med Assoc 2006;228(4):506–10.
33. CDC. West Nile virus: fight the bite! Avoid mosquito bites to avoid infection. Available at: http://www.cdc.gov/ncidod/dvbid/westnile/prevention_info.htm. Accessed June 4, 2008.
34. PFSE. Fight bac! Keep food safe from bacteria. Available at: http://www.fightbac.org/. Accessed June 4, 2008.
35. CDC. Framework for program evaluation in public health. MMWR Recomm Rep 1999;48(RR-11):1–40.
36. Sidwa TJ, Wilson PJ, Moore GM, et al. Evaluation of oral rabies vaccination programs for control of rabies epizootics in coyotes and gray foxes: 1995–2003. J Am Vet Med Assoc 2005;227(5):785–92.

37. Gage KL, Dennis DT, Orloski KA, et al. Cases of cat-associated human plague in the western US, 1977–1998. Clin Infect Dis 2000;30(6):893–900.
38. Blanton JD, Hanlon CA, Rupprecht CE. Rabies surveillance in the United States during 2006. J Am Vet Med Assoc 2007;231(4):540–56.
39. CDC. Mass treatment of humans exposed to rabies—New Hampshire, 1994. MMWR Morb Mortal Wkly Rep 1995;44(26):484–6.
40. APHA. Rickettsiiosis, tickborne: I. Rocky Mountain spotted fever. In: Benenson AS, editor. Control of communicable diseases manual. 16th edition. Washington, DC: American Public Health Association; 1995. p. 401–3.
41. Elchos BN, Goddard J. Implications of presumptive fatal Rocky Mountain spotted fever in two dogs and their owner. J Am Vet Med Assoc 2003;223(10):1450–2, 1433.
42. The Merek veterinary manual—zoonoses: introduction (Table: global zoonoses). Available at: http://www.merckvetmanual.com/mvm/index.jsp%3Fcfile%3Dhtm/bc/220100.htm. Accessed July 17, 2008.
43. Wright JG, Tengelsen LA, Smith KE, et al. Multidrug-resistant Salmonella typhimurium in four animal facilities. Emerging Infect Dis 2005;11(8):1235–41.
44. USDA. Screwworm. Available at: http://www.aphis.usda.gov/lpa/pubs/fsscworm.html. Accessed May 31, 2008.
45. Garris G. Veterinarian averts screwworm outbreak. J Am Vet Med Assoc 1998; 212(2):159.

Disease Reporting and Surveillance: Where Do Companion Animal Diseases Fit In?

George E. Moore, DVM, MS, PhD[a],*, Elizabeth Lund, DVM, MPH, PhD[b]

KEYWORDS

• Surveillance • Disease reporting • Zoonoses
• Databases • Networks

In 1858, Rudolph Virchow, the father of comparative medicine, stated: "Between animal and human medicine there are no dividing lines—nor should there be."[1] People and animals are intimate partners in the world today. Some animals live with us as companions. Others play economic roles as, for example, food producers. Because we live with animals and rely on animals, understanding the impact of disease in animal populations is important. Diseases in animal populations can affect human populations in three ways:

Animals can transmit diseases (zoonoses) to humans (eg, rabies).
Diseases that affect both animals and humans may affect animals more readily or earlier than humans, thus providing an early warning as a sentinel of human risk (eg, West Nile virus).
Diseases in animals can threaten the economic health of the human population, because animals have economic value.[2]

The first two of these ways are the most relevant to public health concerns related to companion animals. A comprehensive public health perspective takes the human-animal interface into consideration through disease surveillance and reporting in animals, including companion animals.

WHAT IS SURVEILLANCE?

The definition of public health surveillance used by the Centers for Disease Control and Prevention is "the ongoing, systematic collection, analysis, and interpretation of

[a] Department of Comparative Pathobiology, School of Veterinary Medicine, Purdue University, 725 Harrison Street, West Lafayette, IN 47907, USA
[b] Banfield, The Pet Hospital, 8000 NE Tillamook, P.O. Box 13998, Portland, OR 97213, USA
* Corresponding author.
E-mail address: gemoore@purdue.edu (G.E. Moore).

Vet Clin Small Anim 39 (2009) 225–240
doi:10.1016/j.cvsm.2008.10.009
0195-5616/08/$ – see front matter © 2009 Elsevier Inc. All rights reserved.
vetsmall.theclinics.com

health-related data essential to the planning, implementation, and evaluation of public health practice, closely integrated with the timely dissemination of these data to those responsible for prevention and control."[3] This definition incorporates the concepts of regular collection of health-related information, an interpretation of this information, and actions by appropriate agencies or individuals based on this "new" information.[4] Although *surveillance* and *monitoring* are sometimes used interchangeably, surveillance is usually considered related to but distinct from monitoring, which is the routine periodic collection of information.[5]

Surveillance for public health purposes has many uses besides those related to detecting outbreaks or estimating the magnitude of a disease or health problem (**Box 1**).[6] Such uses and functions include the facilitation of planning for appropriate interventions and evaluating the effectiveness of control and prevention measures. All uses, however, are influenced by the quality and quantity of information collected.

The collection of health-related information is the foundation and most labor-intensive aspect of public health surveillance. Surveillance systems can be classified as *active* or *passive*. In active surveillance, the health agency or department initiates regular contact with reporting sources (eg, hospitals, clinics, or laboratories). This method increases the likelihood that reporting is complete. However this method has traditionally required a good deal of labor and has been costly to implement.[7] In passive surveillance, the collecting entity relies on individuals at the reporting sources to initiate voluntary reports. Historically, passive surveillance methods have been used much more frequently than active surveillance.

In compensation for its costs, active surveillance is typically timely, relatively complete and accurate, and can produce estimates of disease frequency. However, because active surveillance is so labor intensive, collecting agencies may decide to limit the scope of the geographic area or type of respondents surveyed, which can result in bias. Conversely, passive surveillance systems, with less effort and less cost, may be able to collect information from a much broader geographic or demographic area than an active system. However, passive surveillance systems typically suffer from underreporting or incomplete reporting, have a greater potential for reporting bias, and frequently lack denominator values (the population at risk).

Box 1
Uses of disease surveillance and reporting in public health

Quantitatively estimate the magnitude of a health problem

Portray, in time or space, the natural history of a disease

Document the distribution and spread of a health event

Detect epidemics, or identify a public health problem

Formulate and test hypotheses

Stimulate and facilitate research

Evaluate control and prevention measures

Monitor changes in infectious agents

Detect changes in health practices

Facilitate planning

Data from Thacker SB. Historical development. In: Teutsch SM, Churchill RE, editors. Principles and practice of public health surveillance. 2nd edition. New York: Oxford University Press; 2000. p. 1–16.

Public health agencies often attempt to reduce underreporting in passive surveillance through institution of legal mandates to require reporting of selected diseases. Both because of the lower financial burden to maintain passive surveillance and because of the need for long-term surveillance, most routine notifiable-disease surveillance systems rely on passive reporting.[8] Meanwhile, active surveillance systems are becoming increasingly cost-efficient through improved computer technology, health care networks, and data record linkage. Combinations of active and passive methods are often used now in disease surveillance.

SURVEILLANCE FOR PEOPLE AND ANIMALS

Scientists have noted that, of the nearly 1500 species of infectious organisms known to be pathogenic to humans, more than 60% are zoonotic.[9] An even greater percentage (75%–80%) of emerging pathogens or pathogens likely to be used in bioterrorism are zoonoses.[10] The need to know more about infectious diseases has been an impetus for human disease surveillance, although diseases transmitted from vertebrate animals to humans (ie, zoonoses) have not been a primary focus of these surveillance efforts. Nevertheless, disease surveillance is currently conducted separately for selected diseases of people and of animals by organizations at levels ranging from global to local (**Table 1**). Many hospital-based systems in the United States also seek to capture information for diseases/conditions that are not infectious (eg, toxicologic, environmental, cancer related, related to birth defects).

Global or International

Human
The World Health Organization (WHO), founded in 1948, is the directing and coordinating authority for health within the United Nations system. Headquartered in Geneva, Switzerland, WHO also has six regional offices. Like the United Nations, WHO does

Table 1
Primary organizations involved in disease surveillance

Organization Level	Surveillance Responsibility	
	Human	**Animal**
International/ intergovernmental	World Health Organization	World Organization for Animal Health (formerly Office International des Epizooties)
National/federal	Department of Health and Human Services; Centers for Disease Control and Prevention	Department of Agriculture; Animal Plant Health Inspection Service; Veterinary Service; Centers for Epidemiology and Animal Health; Center for Emerging Issues; National Animal Health Monitoring System; National Surveillance Unit
State	State departments of health	State departments of agriculture, or boards of animal health
Local	County/municipal public health offices	None, or area regulatory veterinarians
Nongovernmental	Corporate, private, or academic hospitals; disease registries	Corporate, private, or academic veterinary hospitals; disease registries or databases

not have enforcement authority over member countries. WHO cannot mandate participation in disease surveillance and relies on passive reporting of disease. A zoonotic disease of great concern to WHO is rabies, with more than 50,000 deaths reported annually around the world. Many of these deaths involve children.[11]

The Pan American Health Organization (PAHO), headquartered in Washington, DC, works to improve health in the countries of the Americas. It also serves as the WHO's regional office for the Americas. PAHO's list of reportable diseases is tailored to those of major concern in the Americas. Many infectious diseases reportable to PAHO and WHO, are arthropod-borne diseases.

Animal

The Office International des Epizooties (OIE), now termed the World Organization for Animal Health, was created in 1924 to fight animal diseases at a global level. The headquarters of OIE is in Paris, France. Although the 2008 list of diseases notifiable to the OIE (http://www.oie.int/eng/maladies/en_classification2008.htm?e1d7) includes diseases of companion animals (eg, rabies, leptospirosis, tularemia, and anthrax), the disease lists are commonly grouped by the large-animal species affected. OIE's recognition by international trade organizations underscores the traditional economic importance of animals, and the negative impact of food-animal diseases, within society. Like WHO, OIE relies on passive surveillance.

National

Human

In the United States, the Centers for Disease Control and Prevention (CDC), in Atlanta, Georgia, under the federal Department of Health and Human Services, has responsibility for the collection and publication of data concerning nationally notifiable infectious diseases. The CDC operates the National Notifiable Diseases Surveillance System (NNDSS: http://www.cdc.gov/ncphi/disss/nndss/nndsshis.htm), through which states report diseases. A list of diseases that should be voluntarily reported by states is determined by representatives from the Council of State and Territorial Epidemiologists, with input from CDC,[8] but reporting is only mandated through individual state legislation or regulation. Data on selected notifiable diseases are published weekly by the CDC in the *Morbidity and Mortality Weekly Report*. Animal rabies data (including cat and dog) are collected from states as part of NNDSS and compiled annually in a summary report.

The CDC also operates several disease surveillance systems that focus on specific diseases or etiologies. These systems include the West Nile Virus Surveillance System, the Foodborne Diseases Active Surveillance Network, and the Waterborne Disease Outbreak Surveillance. These systems, with the exception of that for West Nile virus, only collect and report data for human cases of disease.

Animal

The US Department of Agriculture (USDA) Animal and Plant Health Inspection Service (APHIS) has national responsibility for animal health issues. Within APHIS, Veterinary Services operates the Centers for Epidemiology and Animal Health, which is headquartered in Fort Collins, Colorado. These Centers currently include the Center for Emerging Issues, the National Animal Health Monitoring System, and the National Surveillance Unit (NSU).

The NSU coordinates various aspects of USDA disease surveillance through the overarching National Animal Health Surveillance System (NAHSS; http://www.aphis.usda.gov/vs/nahss/nahss.htm). The goal of the NAHSS is to provide greater protection from endemic, emerging, and foreign animal diseases that could affect United States livestock, poultry, and wildlife populations. The NAHSS develops and enhances surveillance systems for foreign and emerging diseases, for analysis of data from laboratory network reports, and for related Veterinary Services animal health efforts.

One component of the multifaceted NAHSS is the National Animal Health Reporting System (NAHRS). In a joint effort with the US Animal Health Association and the American Association of Veterinary Laboratory Diagnosticians, the National Surveillance Unit receives and disseminates reports from chief state animal health officials for the NAHRS. This system was designed for surveillance of confirmed OIE-reportable diseases in specific commercial livestock, poultry, and aquaculture species in the United States.

State and Local

Human
The United States has approximately 50 state, 10 tribal or territorial, and more than 3000 local and county health departments.[12] As previously noted, disease reporting is mandated through state legislation or regulation. The diseases considered notifiable and the requirements for reporting them vary by state.[13] Surveillance may be conducted by state departments of health (who may have a veterinarian on staff) and by local and county public health departments. The division of responsibility and authority between state and local health departments varies substantially by state. In some states, rabies is the only zoonotic disease required to be reported.[14] State and local agencies still typically rely on passive reporting.

Animal
State agencies, such as departments of agriculture or boards of animal health, are the usual primary recipients of animal disease reports from practitioners. Because of the rising population of companion animals, these agencies increasingly have at least one staff member responsible for disease issues in small animals. Their regulatory concerns are often focused on communicable disease threats from intrastate and interstate movement of animals. These state agencies, however, may not have additional resources to conduct companion-animal disease prevention and control activities at a local level.[15] The limited resources of these agencies have also created a reliance on passive surveillance for diseases.

Hospitals, Registries, and Databases

Human
Because of state-mandated reporting, human hospitals and clinics have been involved in disease surveillance for many years. Likewise numerous registries and databases have been developed, usually independent of each other. As hospitals have progressed to electronic medical records, increasing the speed of data access, disease surveillance has become more integrated with hospital information systems, enabling health care providers to meet the specific reporting requirements for their hospitals and their local and state health departments.

Animal
For many years, the only system that routinely collected medical information about companion-animal disease was the Veterinary Medical database (VMDB) (http://www.vmdb.org), currently housed in Urbana, Illinois. The VMDB was started in 1964 as an initiative of the National Cancer Institute for the purpose of comparative medicine and the study of cancer in companion animals. The VMDB now collects standardized information on all, not just cancer, cases seen at colleges and schools of veterinary

medicine in North America. Case submission, however, is voluntary and many, but not all, universities participate. Another limitation of the VMDB is the lack of impetus for timely reporting, and different institutions lag behind at different rates. Although the VMDB cannot provide timely information for disease surveillance, it could provide valuable historical trends. A strength of the database is the reliability of the information. The information comes from board-certified specialists at university teaching hospitals with an array of diagnostic methods at their disposal, thus giving users confidence in the recorded diagnoses. However, because these institutions typically operate as referral hospitals, conclusions should be formulated carefully, the data needs to be used cautiously, especially when attempting to generalize for some diseases to the larger population seen in primary-care settings.

A FRAGMENTED LANDSCAPE

As noted in the preceding organizational descriptions, disease surveillance occurs at many different levels and for many different purposes. In 2006, a report by a US House of Representatives Committee on Government Reform described the public health surveillance system in America as "a gaudy patchwork of jurisdictionally narrow, wildly variant, technologically backward data collection and communications capabilities."[16] Although this report did not specifically address animal-disease surveillance methods, disease surveillance for human health and for animal health is typically and traditionally separate from the global scale down to the local level. As already described, because authority related to such surveillance is delegated to the states in the United States, states vary widely in their reporting requirements for zoonotic diseases in terms of the specific diseases to be reported and the level or agency to receive the report. The policies for farm animals, companion animals, wildlife, and human health often fail to intersect. As various agencies pursue their mandates, there are no comprehensive laws or approaches to monitor, report on, or manage companion-animal zoonoses.[17] A National Academy of Sciences report, while not focusing on diseases solely of companion animals, has proposed a coordinated mechanism for improving collaboration and cooperation among local, state, and federal agencies, and the private sector health community for improved animal-disease surveillance.[18] It remains to be determined who will take the lead on this proposal, or how it will receive funding and support for coordinating activities.

As noted by the National Academy of Sciences report, the landscape in disease surveillance is fragmented. Limitations that undermine organizational capacities include:[17]

Gaps in regulatory authority
Lack of enforcement capacity for some authorities
Unequal distribution of resources among health-related sectors and agencies
Less-than-optimal communication and resource sharing, including data incompatibility, across relevant sectors and agencies
Competition among sectors and agencies for limited resources
Lack of adequate scientific and socioeconomic data for informed regulatory decisions
Significant time lags in authority enactment and thus inability of most agencies to enact rapid response measures

REPORTING, SURVEILLANCE, AND INFORMATION SYSTEMS

In public health, there are generally three types of notifiable disease reports: (1) individual case reports with information captured on each diseased individual; (2) reports that present aggregated data on the total number of individuals with the disease or conditions; and (3) more detailed reports on the total number of cases or syndromes when an outbreak or public health emergency is suspected.[7] Each type of report generally requires the collection of specific information, often facilitated by the use of standardized forms.

Our capacity to manage medical information (termed *medical informatics*) has exponentially improved because of technologic advances in the last few decades. The increasingly widespread use of personal computers in public health has led to the development of many information systems that can support surveillance and health-related information. However, these systems operate as stand-alone systems without record sharing. Nevertheless, continuous advancements in informatics technology will continue to result in increased availability of information, improved methods to collect and disseminate data, greater potential for real-time access to data, and increased opportunity for data sharing.

Computerized entry of clinical and laboratory data at the point of care is becoming more common in health care, as this method improves timeliness, legibility, and accessibility of medical information.[19] Additionally, with electronic data security, Internet-based applications are increasingly used by clinicians, staff, laboratories, and health departments for entering or collecting health data.[20]

Electronic records ideally maintain better data quantity, quality, and interpretability as compared with traditional paper medical records, while concurrently improving the speed of data access and analysis. Entries in disease reports and medical records typically contain many concepts that can and should be incorporated into an information system and relational database (**Table 2**).[21] Advances in technology also allow records from two or more sources that contain different types of information to be linked into a single file for an individual. Integrating or linking data across data sources can provide more robust information for testing hypotheses or for assessing prevention and control activities. For example, linkage of a patient's pharmacy prescription data and clinical pathology test data could be used to investigate if alterations in clinical chemistry tests were associated with new medication use or possible interaction of medications. Data linkages have also highlighted the need to ensure computer system compatibility, availability of accurate linkage information, and establish procedures to resolve data discrepancies.[7]

Proprietary or "stand-alone" systems work against the integration of health information. To promote integration of health-related information, including laboratory data, disease surveillance systems must use standardized classification systems.[22,23] Although not comprehensive in human medicine, standardized classification systems do exist for electronic message structure (Health Level 7), for causes of morbidity or death (eg, *International Statistical Classification of Disease, 10th Revision [ICD-10]*), for clinical laboratory result reporting (eg, Logical Observation and Identifier Names and Codes), and for medical and pathology findings (Systematized Nomenclature of Medicine [SNOMED]).[24] An initiative of the National Library of Medicine, the Unified Medical Language System is a linked collection of vocabularies from the biomedical sciences that enables translation between systems of standardized terminology, like SNOMED, to be used for health data aggregation and information, as well as for informatics research (http://www.nlm.nih.gov/research/umls/).

For reporting standards, no veterinary diagnostic codes in widespread use are comparable to the *ICD-10* codes for human disease. An attempt to create the Standardized Nomenclature for Veterinary Medicine (SNOVET), linked to SNOMED, was begun in the 1970s but has not been sustained. The Standardized Nomenclature for Veterinary Disease and Operations (SNVDO) has also been developed, but is only

Table 2
Concepts coded in disease reports and health care information systems

Name	Example
Diagnoses	Tularemia
Species	Feline
Breed	DSH
Date of birth (or age)	mm/dd/yyyy
Date of death	mm/dd/yyyy
Sex/neuter status	Male castrated
Weight (unit)	3.4 kg
Address	Hospital, owner, or farm address
Date of report/observation	mm/dd/yyyy
Human/animal contacts and # ill	H/A contacts: 1/0; ill:0/0
Clinical signs	Fever
Laboratory tests	ALT, GGT
Laboratory result	(Number)
Units of measure	IU/L
Disease-causing organism	*Francisella tularensis*
Histopathology/cytology result	Granulomatous inflammation
Surgical/invasive procedures	Fine needle aspirate
Anatomic sites	Lymph node—prescapular
Drugs/therapeutics	Gentamicin
Drug regimens	5 mg/kg q24hr × 10 days SC
Outcome measures	Died

Abbreviations: ALT, alanine aminotransferase; DSH, domestic shorthair; GGT, gamma glutamyl transpeptidase; H/A, human/animal; SC, subcutaneous.

Data from McDonald CJ, Overhage JM, Dexter P, et al. A framework for capturing clinical data sets from computerized sources. Ann Intern Med 1997;127:675–82.

used in some systems (eg, VMDB). A significant proportion of SNDVO codes cannot be mapped to a SNOMED concept,[25,26] prompting further initiatives toward improved methods in coding. A system of standardized nomenclature for private companion-animal practice, PetTerms, has been developed by the University of Minnesota to facilitate the collection of epidemiologic data on dogs and cats seen in private veterinary practice.[27] In addition, the American Animal Hospital Association, as part of an electronic health record initiative, is currently developing standardized diagnostic terms, including a microglossary of SNOMED terms, to use in companion-animal practice.[28] Nevertheless, compared with human medicine, veterinary medicine lacks the regulatory or financial drivers to ensure that these critical informatics components are developed and implemented.

Changes in veterinary practice, practice management, and electronic medical record systems are providing valuable new resources that increase our capacity to conduct companion-animal disease surveillance. Despite these efforts, limited development and adoption of standardized medical nomenclature remains a major impediment to both integrated animal-disease surveillance and integrated public health surveillance. Nevertheless, surveillance and other information systems continue to be developed privately and commercially, sometimes with and sometimes without concerted efforts for compatibility and interoperability.

EVALUATING PUBLIC HEALTH SURVEILLANCE SYSTEMS

Twenty years ago, the CDC published *Guidelines for Evaluating Surveillance Systems* to promote the best use of public health resources. The integration of health information systems and the electronic exchange of health data, among other factors, prompted an update to these *Guidelines* in 2001.[29] The *Guidelines* provide nine system attributes (**Table 3**) that can be assessed as part of an overall system evaluation. Such attributes should also be considered for any system used in companion-animal disease surveillance.

Simplicity

Surveillance systems should be as simple as possible while still capable of meeting the system's objectives. This simplicity should be evident from the user interface for data entry through the analysis phase and the generation of reports.

Acceptability

This simplicity can also affect the system's acceptability by participants and end-users. Also related to system acceptability are the objectives of the surveillance and costs/benefits of participation. Reduced acceptability can affect reporting rates, timeliness of reporting, and completeness of reports.[30,31]

Flexibility

A flexible surveillance system can adapt to changing needs with little additional time, personnel, or allocated funds. This flexibility is important when considering the addition of diseases, data streams, or information technology.

Stability

Changes to the flexibility of a surveillance system can also affect its stability (ie, reliability for timely data collection, management, and analysis).

Table 3 Important attributes of disease surveillance systems	
Attribute	**Meaning**
Simplicity	Simple structure and easy operation
Acceptability	Strong willingness of persons and organizations to participate
Flexibility	High level of adaptability to changing information needs or operating conditions
Stability	Good operational reliability and ready availability of system
Timeliness	Short intervals between steps in surveillance
Data quality	High levels of completeness and validity of data
Representativeness	Reported events highly typical for larger population in terms of time, place, and patient
Sensitivity	High proportion of disease cases detected by system
Predictive value positive	High proportion of reported cases that actually have the disease of interest

Data from Schultz K. AAHA developing unified diagnostic code to improve care. DVM Newsmagazine 2007;11:1S. Available at: http://www.dvmnews.com/dvm/article/articleDetail.jsp?id=475597. Accessed June 24, 2008.

Timeliness

Even in the absence of a perceived disease threat, timeliness of reporting is important. Disease prevention and control, as a goal of surveillance, requires information dissemination in time to "make a difference" (ie, curtail an outbreak). Factors potentially affecting timeliness in surveillance include, but are not limited to, availability of health care facilities and providers, symptom or disease recognition, time required for disease testing and laboratory reporting, and time until confirmed diagnoses are entered by the attending clinician. Nevertheless, with electronic data capture in hospitals and laboratories, some systems are attempting to target "near real-time" surveillance and detection of disease. Because timeliness is a key performance measure in public health surveillance, methods have been developed in recent years to evaluate the effectiveness of systems to provide timely notification of disease outbreaks.[32,33]

Data Quality

Increasing use of electronic data collection and data interchange has increased user expectations and can improve timeliness, but it doesn't obviate the need for validation of captured data. Thus, data quality is critical to the success of any surveillance system. Data quality is determined by complete collection of all variables of interest and standardized data entry (eg, abbreviations and codes) for easy retrieval and analysis. Standardized coding (eg, SNOVET) that is used in some veterinary systems may not be relational with coding in other public health systems (eg, *International Classification of Diseases, Ninth Revision* codes). Other coding methods may be proprietary to the designer or commercial application being used. Data entries must accurately convey information, such as the demographic characteristics, of the patient or survey subjects, the health event of interest (including clinical signs, laboratory tests, diagnostic procedures, diagnoses, therapeutics, and concomitant illnesses or medications), and important risk factors or confounding variables. Although a full assessment of validity may require a special study,[34] reviews of the data and results from studies using the system provide an indication of the relative validity of the collected data.

Representativeness

Systems often collect information from a limited (sample) population with inferences then made to a larger target population. Such inferences are based on an assumption of representativeness. Passive surveillance systems often have widespread access, but, as mentioned, suffer from underreporting or biases in reporting. Systems that are hospital-based typically collect information from all their patients but are closed to data entry from other groups. Differential reporting among different population subgroups can lead to incorrect conclusions related to risk or characterization (eg, severity) of the disease.[35,36] Complete and valid data are critical to assessing the representativeness of the collected information relative to actual events. An accurate assessment of representativeness is difficult, however, if the true characteristics of the larger (eg, national) population are not known.

Sensitivity

In addition to all the aforementioned attributes, a surveillance system must be sensitive, which is determined by the capability to identify an appropriate proportion of the health events of interest. The sensitivity of a system, however, is often influenced by factors independent of the technical structure of the system. Disease identification can be affected by the rate of disease occurrence, the likelihood of a patient entering the health care system using surveillance, and the clinical acumen and testing resources of the medical professionals responsible for reporting cases.

Predictive Value Positive

Some systems seek to improve timeliness and sensitivity by collecting case information before confirmation of the suspected diagnosis. Public health response, however, is ideally founded on a high proportion of reported cases that actually have the disease under surveillance—the predictive value positive (PVP).[37] A system with low PVP for a health event can result in incorrect communication pertaining to the event and in misdirected resources. As an indicator of false-positive reports, the PVP may also point toward larger problems in data validity and, ultimately, in acceptability of the system.

USING NEW DATA SOURCES IN COMPANION-ANIMAL DISEASE SURVEILLANCE

Surveillance of animal diseases for public health purposes, as already noted, may be justified because animals, for certain diseases, are more readily affected or are affected earlier than are humans. Animals have therefore been considered "sentinels" for human disease (eg, canary in the mine). Not surprisingly, the value of animals as sentinels or the basis of a sentinel surveillance system may be effective for some diseases (eg, West Nile virus),[38] but not others, such as nonzoonotic infections or selected toxins.[39]

Public health surveillance, however, in recent years has applied the term *sentinel surveillance system* to surveillance from selected sources (eg, infectious disease practitioners).[13,40] Veterinarians should therefore be aware that such terminology can be used without requiring (or even considering) the use of animals or animal diseases for surveillance.

Hospitals and Hospital Groups

Diagnostic surveillance

Although many university veterinary hospitals have provided diagnoses and related data to the VMDB for many years, the small number of submitting hospitals (<30 in North America), the uniqueness of the referral patient population, and the timeliness of data submission present marked limitations in disease surveillance. Some private and corporate practices in the United States, however, now have tens, or even hundreds, of hospital locations and provide primary care to thousands, or even millions, of patients annually. Although such large numbers of locations and patients are extremely valuable for surveillance, medical information from different locations must be linked, in compatible language, and accessible (via networks or permissions).

One such large practice is Banfield, The Pet Hospital, headquartered in Portland, Oregon. All Banfield hospital locations (>700) use a proprietary electronic medical records system called PetWare, developed by the parent company.[41] Data from all hospital locations are pulled daily into a centralized searchable database, providing an accessible and timely resource of several million small-animal medical records. The potential capabilities were recognized in 2003 when the CDC funded a 2-year project for Purdue University and Banfield to collaboratively use this very large companion-animal database for public health surveillance.[42] Although the value of this resource has been demonstrated, continued federal funding was not provided to sustain ongoing surveillance for public health purposes.

Syndromic surveillance

Individual clinical signs (eg, fever) may be nonspecific for disease etiology, but an aggregate or "constellation" of signs (ie, a syndrome) may indicate or heighten suspicion of particular diseases. Syndromic surveillance is a new method of surveillance that monitors the frequency and distribution of health-related signs or symptoms, or trends in health care, among a population in a specific geographic area. Syndromic surveillance systems are designed to detect anomalous increases in certain syndromes (eg, skin rashes). These systems can also track potential indicators (eg, increased selected over-the-counter medication sales) that may signal a pre-emergent disease outbreak.[13] Because these systems monitor symptoms and other signs of disease outbreaks early, instead of waiting for clinically confirmed reports or diagnoses of disease, some experts believe that syndromic surveillance systems help public health officials improve timeliness in identifying outbreaks.

Concerns about this approach to surveillance have been raised,[43] as syndromic surveillance systems are resource intensive, are costly to maintain, often require data linkage, and, because of their sensitivity, are more likely than traditional systems to issue false alarms. A rigorous evaluation has not been conducted to demonstrate that these systems can prospectively detect disease or events more rapidly than they would otherwise be detected through traditional surveillance. A retrospective review suggests, however, that the sensitivity and timeliness of syndromic surveillance systems are comparable to or better than diagnosis-based data systems for detecting large seasonally occurring outbreaks.[35] Syndromic surveillance methods have been applied retrospectively to companion-animal records in a large veterinary practice database for the investigation of community exposure to industrial chemicals.[44]

Laboratory-Based Surveillance Networks

Federal- or state-supported laboratories

The CDC and the USDA are working with two national laboratory associations to enhance coordination of zoonotic disease surveillance by adding veterinary diagnostic laboratories to the CDC's Laboratory Response Network.[13] The Laboratory Response Network is an integrated network of public health and clinical laboratories coordinated by the CDC to test specimens and develop diagnostic tests for identifying infectious diseases and biological and chemical weapons. Federal- and state-supported laboratories serve as important resources for notifiable and zoonotic disease information, and they often have well-established communication with other governmental or regulatory organizations. They are typically limited, however, in either the geographic area they serve or the frequency in which practicing veterinarians send them samples for diagnosis.

Corporate or private laboratories

Many veterinarians rely on commercial diagnostic laboratories for prompt pickup, delivery, and testing of diagnostic samples and specimens from their patients. Reporting of test results is often available online through secure access by the veterinarian or clinic staff. These laboratories may be corporately or privately owned, and may be composed of a network of integrated veterinary diagnostic laboratories. They offer a varied range of diagnostic services, but patient information (eg, signalment, history, and clinical signs) associated with the sample or specimen is usually limited.

Nevertheless, the large geographic area of service and number of submissions make veterinary laboratory databases a rich source of information for surveillance. In the United States, the two largest commercial laboratories servicing veterinary practices are Antech Diagnostics, Inc., headquartered in Santa Monica, California, and IDEXX Laboratories, Inc., with United States headquarters in Westbrook, Maine. Veterinary laboratory databases have already been used to investigate the epidemiology of infectious diseases using serologic[45,46] and microbiologic[47] test results.

Internet-Based, or Virtual, Surveillance

The Internet is revolutionizing communications as the electronic network that people anywhere in the world can use to rapidly exchange information. The speed and increasingly common access enable individuals and companies to easily collect reports or conduct surveys, including information related to companion-animal diseases.[48] The ease of data dissemination and data gathering may be offset, however, by biases in reporting.

Surveillance for infectious disease outbreaks affecting, or potentially affecting, companion animals can be found on ProMED-mail (http://www.promedmail.org). ProMED (Program for Monitoring Emerging Diseases) is an electronic outbreak reporting system that monitors infectious diseases globally, collecting information for dissemination to subscribers. ProMED-mail is a moderated e-mail list, and subscribers can receive new postings based on their indicated interests. ProMED-mail is developed and maintained by the International Society for Infectious Diseases. Other initiatives have been developed to search and "score" Internet-based communications, such as ProMED, and then report pertinent changes in frequency, severity, or geography for selected infectious diseases.[49]

ROLE OF VETERINARY MEDICAL ASSOCIATIONS AND GROUPS

Several professional organizations in veterinary medicine are composed of individuals with interest and expertise in public health (**Table 4**). Even though these organizations do not typically control personnel or financial assets to conduct disease surveillance, they are stakeholders in the conduct of such surveillance and have members who are subject-matter experts in this area. Although many individuals with expertise in public health surveillance do not currently have experience in companion-animal practice, this number will undoubtedly increase in the future. Such organizations and individuals who interface with human public health must also champion a "one medicine" concept that considers the role of companion animals in zoonotic disease transmission, as sentinels, and in comparative medicine. These organizations also serve as valuable resources and points of contact for practicing veterinarians with questions about

Table 4
Veterinary professional organizations that can provide contacts or information pertaining to public health and companion-animal disease reporting

Organization	Abbreviation	Web Site
National Association of State Public Health Veterinarians	NASPHV	http://www.nasphv.org
American College of Veterinary Preventive Medicine	ACVPM	http://www.acvpm.org
American Association of Public Health Veterinarians	AAPHV	No Web site
Association for Veterinary Epidemiology and Preventive Medicine	AVEPM	http://www.cvm.uiuc.edu/avepm/
American Veterinary Medical Association	AVMA	http://www.avma.org

companion-animal disease reporting. Dr. Calvin Schwabe's vision a quarter-century ago of "one medicine," in which human and veterinary medicine work together to protect the public health,[50] has never been more relevant.

SUMMARY

Disease surveillance and reporting is a necessary and integral part of public health practice. Although surveillance systems have been developed over many years in human and veterinary medicine, these systems are not usually interconnected. In our current information technology age, the development and integration of existing and new resources in companion-animal practice should be focused on "one medicine—one health" for the betterment and health of all species.

REFERENCES

1. Klauder JV. Interrelations of human and veterinary medicine. N Engl J Med 1958; 258:170–7.
2. Shephard R, Aryel RM, Shaffer L. Animal health. In: Wagner MM, Moore AW, Aryel RM, editors. Handbook of biosurveillance. Boston: Elsevier Academic Press; 2006. p. 111–27.
3. Centers for Disease Prevention and Control. Public health surveillance. Available at: http://www.cdc.gov/ncphi/disss/nndss/phs/overview.htm. Accessed April 20, 2008.
4. Thacker SB, Berkelman RL. Public health surveillance in the United States. Epidemiol Rev 1988;10:164–90.
5. Thrusfield M. Veterinary epidemiology. 3rd edition. Ames (IA): Blackwell Science Ltd.; 2005.
6. Thacker SB. Historical development. In: Teutsch SM, Churchill RE, editors. Principles and practice of public health surveillance. 2nd edition. New York: Oxford University Press; 2000. p. 1–16.
7. Groseclose SL, Sullivan KM, Gibbs NP, et al. Management of the surveillance information system and quality control of data. In: Teutsch SM, Churchill RE, editors. Principles and practice of public health surveillance. New York: Oxford University Press; 2000. p. 95–111.
8. Teutsch SM. Considerations in planning a surveillance system. In: Teutsch SM, Churchill RE, editors. Principles and practice of public health surveillance. 2nd edition. New York: Oxford University Press; 2000. p. 17–29.
9. Taylor LH, Latham SM, Woolhouse ME. Risk factors for human disease emergence. Philos Trans R Soc Lond, B, Biol Sci 2001;356:983–9.
10. Franz DR, Jahrling PB, Friedlander AM, et al. Clinical recognition and management of patients exposed to biological warfare agents. JAMA 1997;278:399–411.
11. Who. Rabies. Available at: http://www.who.int/mediacentre/factsheets/fs099/en/. Accessed May 14, 2008.
12. Velikina R, Dato V, Wagner MM. Governmental public health. In: Wagner MM, Moore AW, Aryel RM, editors. Handbook of biosurveillance. Boston: Elsevier Academic Press; 2006. p. 67–87.
13. Emerging infectous diseases: review of state and federal disease surveillance efforts. GAO-04-877 Report to US Senate Committee. Washington, DC: United States Government Accounting Office, 2004.
14. Wohl JS, Nusbaum KE. Public health roles for small animal practitioners. J Am Vet Med Assoc 2007;230:494–500.

15. Kahn LH. Confronting zoonoses, linking human and veterinary medicine. Emerg Infect Dis 2006;12:556–61.
16. US Congress House of Representatives Committee on Government Reform. Strengthening disease surveillance: eighth report. Washington, DC: US Government Printing Office; 2006.
17. Reaser JK, Clark EE Jr, Meyers NM. All creatures great and minute: a public policy primer for companion animal zoonoses. Zoonoses Public Health 2008; 55:385–401.
18. National Research Council. Animal health at the crossroads: preventing, detecting, and diagnosing animal diseases. Washington, DC: National Academies Press; 2005.
19. Shortliffe EH. The evolution of electronic medical records. Acad Med 1999;74: 414–9.
20. Ward LD, Spain CV, Perilla MJ, et al. Improving disease reporting by clinicians: the effect of an internet-based intervention. J Public Health Manag Pract 2008; 14:56–61.
21. McDonald CJ, Overhage JM, Dexter P, et al. A framework for capturing clinical data sets from computerized sources. Ann Intern Med 1997;127:675–82.
22. Bell PD. Standards and the integrated electronic health care record. Health Care Manag (Frederick) 2000;19:39–43.
23. Sloane EB, Carey CC. Using standards to automate electronic health records (EHRs) and to create integrated healthcare enterprises. Conf Proc IEEE Eng Med Biol Soc 2007;2007:6178–9.
24. Pinner RW. Public health surveillance and information technology. Emerg Infect Dis 1998;4:462–4.
25. Folk LC, Hahn AW, Patrick TB, et al. Salvaging legacy data: mapping an obsolete medical nomenclature to a modern one. Biomed Sci Instrum 2002;38: 405–10.
26. Wurtz RM, Popovich ML. In: Animal disease surveillance: a framework for supporting disease detection in public health, vol. 2008. Scientific Technologies Corporation; 2002.
27. Lund EM, Klausner JS, Ellis LB, et al. PetTerms: a standardized nomenclature for companion animal practice. Online J Vet Res 1998;2:64–86. Available at: http://www.cpb.ouhsc.edu/ojvr/pettermsabs.htm. Accessed June 16, 2008.
28. Schultz K. AAHA developing unified diagnostic code to improve care. DVM Newsmagazine 2007 November 1. Available at: http://www.dvmnews.com/dvm/article/articleDetail.jsp?id=475597. Accessed June 24, 2008.
29. Centers for Disease Control and Prevention. Updated guidelines for evaluating public health surveillance systems. Recommendations from the Guidelines Working Group. MMWR Recomm Rep 2001;50(RR-13):1–35.
30. Sosin DM. Draft framework for evaluating syndromic surveillance systems. J Urban Health 2003;80(Suppl 1):i8–13.
31. Allport R, Mosha R, Bahari M, et al. The use of community-based animal health workers to strengthen disease surveillance systems in Tanzania. Rev Sci Tech 2005;24:921–32.
32. Jajosky RA, Groseclose SL. Evaluation of reporting timeliness of public health surveillance systems for infectious diseases. BMC Public Health 2004;4: 29–37.
33. Dausey DJ, Lurie N, Diamond A, et al. Tests to evaluate public health reporting systems in local public health agencies. Santa Monica (CA): RAND Corporation; 2005.

34. Mucci LA, Wood PA, Cohen B, et al. Validity of self-reported health plan information in a population-based health survey. J Public Health Manag Pract 2006;12: 570–7.
35. Buckeridge DL. Outbreak detection through automated surveillance: a review of the determinants of detection. J Biomed Inform 2007;40:370–9.
36. Bax R, Bywater R, Cornaglia G, et al. Surveillance of antimicrobial resistance–what, how and whither? Clin Microbiol Infect 2001;7:316–25.
37. German RR. Sensitivity and predictive value positive measurements for public health surveillance systems. Epidemiology 2000;11:720–7.
38. Eidson M, Komar N, Sorhage F, et al. Crow deaths as a sentinel surveillance system for West Nile virus in the northeastern United States. Emerg Infect Dis 1999; 2001(7):615–20.
39. Rabinowitz P, Wiley J, Odofin L, et al. Animals as sentinels of chemical terrorism agents: an evidence-based review. Clin Toxicol (Phila) 2008;46:93–100.
40. The emerging infections network: a new venture for the Infectious Diseases Society of America. Executive committee of the infectious diseases society of America emerging infections network. Clin Infect Dis 1997;25:34–6.
41. Faunt K, Lund E, Novak W. The power of practice: harnessing patient outcomes for clinical decision making. Vet Clin North Am Small Anim Pract 2007;37:521–32.
42. Glickman LT, Moore GE, Glickman NW, et al. Purdue University-Banfield National Companion Animal Surveillance Program for emerging and zoonotic diseases. Vector Borne Zoonotic Dis 2006;6:14–23.
43. Reingold A. If syndromic surveillance is the answer, what is the question? Biosecur Bioterror 2003;1:77–81.
44. Maciejewski R, Glickman N, Moore G, et al. Companion animals as sentinels for community exposure to industrial chemicals: the Fairburn, GA, propyl mercaptan case study. Public Health Rep 2008;123:333–42.
45. Moore GE, Guptill LF, Glickman NW, et al. Canine leptospirosis, United States, 2002–2004. Emerg Infect Dis 2006;12:501–3.
46. Miller RI, Ross SP, Sullivan ND, et al. Clinical and epidemiological features of canine leptospirosis in North Queensland. Aust Vet J 2007;85:13–9.
47. Rich M, Deighton L, Roberts L. Clindamycin-resistance in methicillin-resistant Staphylococcus aureus isolated from animals. Vet Microbiol 2005;111:237–40.
48. Gobar GM, Case JT, Kass PH. Program for surveillanceof causes of death of dogs, using the Internet to survey small animal practitioners. J Am Vet Med Assoc 1998;213:215–56.
49. Mykhaloskiy E, Weir L. The Global Public Health Intelligence Network and early warning outbreak detection: a Canadian contribution to global public health. Can J Public Health 2006;97:42–4.
50. Schwabe CW. The challenge of "one medicine:" implications for veterinary practice. In: Veterinary medicine and human health. Baltimore (MD): Williams & Wilkins; 1984. p. 1–15.

Companion Animals as Sentinels for Public Health

Peggy L. Schmidt, DVM, MS[a,b,*]

KEYWORDS

- Surveillance • Veterinary medicine • Infectious disease
- Environmental contamination • Feed contamination
- Bioterrorism

The concept of using animals as sentinels for danger is not new. From the domestication of dogs to protect and warn of impending danger to the introduction of canaries in coal mines, people have used animals to protect health. While archeologists continue to debate about when dogs were domesticated, their use early on as an early warning system for invading animals or people is generally accepted. Dogs served not only as a warning system to allow extra time to prepare for attack, but also as protectors themselves who joined in the defense against invaders.

In the past century, miners used companion birds as sentinels for environmental hazards in the deep shafts of coal mines. With their rapid heart rates, canaries are more susceptible than humans to the effects of carbon monoxide poisoning or depletion of oxygen. These characteristics made canaries good sentinels for dangerous air quality.[1] If a canary dropped from its perch in the cage, miners quickly exited the area in search of better air. This early warning spared the lives of miners. As for the canaries, they often could be resuscitated and returned to sentinel service another day.[1] Today the phrase "a canary in a coal mine" remains a popular expression for a small misfortune as a harbinger of a much larger disaster.

SENTINEL-ANIMAL SURVEILLANCE

Disease surveillance refers to an active system of collection, analysis, and interpretation of data on health-related conditions. The dissemination of these data is necessary for the planning and implementation of useful public health actions. Sentinel-animal surveillance involves collecting data on disease occurrence in animal populations, which can be used for identification of disease outbreaks, for testing effectiveness

[a] College of Veterinary Medicine, Western University of Health Sciences, 309 E. Second Street, Pomona, CA 91766-1854, USA
[b] School of Public Health, University of Minnesota, Minneapolis, MN, USA
* Corresponding author. College of Veterinary Medicine, Western University of Health Sciences, 309 E. Second Street, Pomona, CA 91766-1854, USA.
E-mail address: pschmidt@westernu.edu

Vet Clin Small Anim 39 (2009) 241–250
doi:10.1016/j.cvsm.2008.10.010
0195-5616/08/$ – see front matter © 2009 Elsevier Inc. All rights reserved.
vetsmall.theclinics.com

of preventive medicine or intervention programs, or for hypothesis testing involving the epidemiology of pathogen.[2] Use of sentinels also provides information on changes in the incidence of a disease over time, geographic spread of disease, and risk factors of specific diseases or syndromes in reference to a specific target population.

Animal sentinels for disease surveillance may be individuals or populations of animals that exhibit particular characteristics. First, the animal must be susceptible to the disease of interest. Sentinels should be just as likely, if not more likely, to be affected by the disease than the target species. Increased susceptibility may allow for early detection, which in turn allows for rapid implementation of disease-control and prevention strategies to avoid or minimize spread of disease in the target species. Second, the animal must generate a measurable clinical or immunologic disease response. Clinical signs of disease should be recognizable in the sentinel, but do not need to be identical to clinical signs of disease in the target species. Immunologic responses should be rapid and easily measured. In routine sampling, points at which seroconversion occurs provide temporal data for assessment of transmission risk. Beyond these two traits, sentinels ideally should pose little risk of zoonotic transmission to people handling the animals and should not contribute to the amplification and spread of the agent as a reservoir. Animal species vary greatly in approaching these ideal characteristics.[3]

Animals can serve as incidental or intentional (or experimental) sentinels for disease. Incidental animal sentinels are not purposefully placed in a situation where disease may occur specifically for the purpose of detection. For instance, animals using the same tap water as their owners serve as incidental sentinels for water-borne illness. Meanwhile, animals sharing a common household environment with their owners serve as incidental sentinels for household environmental contaminants. Conversely, intentional animal sentinels are purposefully placed in areas of potential risk to determine presence of disease. In some instances, intentional sentinels may be selected for their immunologic naiveté to the disease of concern, such as unvaccinated or specific-pathogen–free animals. In other instances, intentional sentinels may immunocompetent animals undergoing routine monitoring for clinical signs or immunologic evidence of disease.

Animal-sentinel systems can range from simple to complex. An example of a simple animal-sentinel system is the classic canary in a coal mine. Pathology laboratory reports of findings on submitted necropsies are also examples of simple animal-sentinel systems. More complex systems may combine incidental and intentionally placed animals, multiple species of sentinels, and advanced diagnostics, such as DNA sequencing and databasing of phylogentic information. Geographic Information Systems mapping and instantaneous global communications have made complex systems of animal sentinels useful on a larger scale.

ANIMAL SENTINELS IN PRODUCTION SETTINGS

In animal-production settings, unvaccinated or immunologically naïve animals are intentionally comingled with the vaccinated population as a means of detecting circulating pathogens within the population. For example, swine veterinarians use unvaccinated pigs to monitor for evidence of remaining circulating porcine reproductive and respiratory syndrome virus (PRRSV) following an outbreak within a production facility.[4,5] Following a PRRSV outbreak, vaccination of the population is implemented in conjunction with other control measures, such as test and cull or herd closure. Once infection is believed to be controlled, seronegative sentinel animals are placed within the population of vaccinated animals. Serum samples are collected from these sentinels at predetermined intervals and tested to detect seroconversion to PRRSV, which would indicate ongoing disease transmission within the population. In worst-case scenarios, the sentinels succumb to PRRSV and confirmation of infection occurs upon necropsy. No matter whether the sentinel survives or dies, the animal provides information about the risk to other members of the population and allows for disease-control and -prevention strategies to be maintained or altered as needed.

Sentinel animals in production settings can also serve as components of more complex public health surveillance efforts. Recent emergence of highly pathogenic avian influenza (HPAI) H5N1 has prompted global efforts to map and predict geographic spread of the disease. Poultry serve as important sentinels for HPAI incursion and spread and have been used to describe the ecology of HPAI outbreaks throughout the world.[6–8] Despite the important role poultry play in HPAI detection, they do posses undesirable characteristics for HPAI sentinels. Poultry are a reservoir species for both low-pathogen avian influenza (LPAI) and HPAI and demonstrate a high risk for zoonotic transmission to animal handlers. Waterfowl in the wild or used in production settings are also naturally susceptible to HPAI infection and have sentinel use, but are more likely to reflect nonlocal disease transmission, either through migration or contact with migrating birds, and are more susceptible to virus mutation than poultry are.[9] Similar to waterfowl, domestic production pigs are susceptible to HPAI and can demonstrate serologic responses to infection, making them another potential production-animal sentinel.[10] However, as with poultry and waterfowl, pigs have the potential to serve as HPAI reservoirs and may pose a risk for zoonotic transmission to animal handlers. Due to the close association between production animals and people, these species rarely serve as intentional sentinels for zoonotic disease. However, they often serve as incidental sentinels for zoonotic disease in public health surveillance.

WILDLIFE SENTINEL SETTINGS

Wildlife serve as classic sentinels for environmental human health risks, as they share the same air, water, and land resources with people. Biological processes of many wildlife species often react to environmental toxins with clinical and pathologic signs that parallel the effects in people. Monitoring wildlife in situ provides integrated data on the type, amount, and bioavailability of contaminants and the clinical effects of exposure. Disease monitoring in wildlife species has permitted the exploration of increases in the incidence of disease syndromes, such as metabolic, endocrine, or reproductive diseases. The resulting findings have generated hypotheses about potential toxins and assisted with the identification of environmental contaminants that pose a risk to human health. For example, examinations of free-living birds (including bald eagles, gulls, terns, and tree swallows), mammals (including mink, river otters, and beluga whales), fish (including walleye, bullheads, and suckers), and amphibians (including snapping turtles and mudpuppies) over multiple decades have revealed numerous human health hazards, such as the contamination of the Great Lakes–St. Lawrence basin of the United States and Canada with dichlorodiphenyltrichloroethane (DDT), polychlorinated biphenyls (PCBs), and dioxin.[11]

COMPANION-ANIMAL SENTINEL SETTINGS

Through interactions with individual patients, veterinarians monitor the health of the animal populations the practices serve. Many diseases seen daily in veterinary practices have the potential to affect the health of animal owners, clinic employees, and community members.

Cats and dogs have been identified as potential sentinels for numerous diseases that also affect people. Companion animals are effective sentinels, as they share a common environment with their owners. In intimate contact with members of the human family, companion animals often eat similar foods, share the same beds, and serve as travel companions, making their disease risk similar to that of their owners. Thus, the health of the companion animal often mirrors the health of or suggests the health risks to humans in the same household. The following examples highlight just a few specific situations where companion animals can serve as sentinels for both animal and human health.

Feed Contamination

Recently, dogs and cats became incidental sentinels for possible contamination in the United States food supply. In March 2007, pet food manufacturer Menu Foods began the first of many recalls of pet food products following increased reports by veterinarians of dogs and cats with renal failure.[12] Other pet food companies soon followed suit, recalling millions of pounds of cat and dog food containing melamine-contaminated wheat gluten that had been imported from China. Unfortunately, many pigs and chickens destined for human consumption were exposed to contaminated feed before the source of contamination could be identified and pulled from the animal food supply.[13] While there were no reports of human illness associated this incident, the massive public attention to the untimely illness and death of pets has led to increased monitoring of imported food supplies for both pets and people.

Infectious Diseases

Many bacteria, viruses, parasites, and fungi infect both companion animals and people. Differences in infectious dose, severity of clinical signs, and immunologic response to infection can lead to detection of some diseases in companion animals before detection in their owners, an important characteristic of a good sentinel. Companion animals are less than ideal as intentional sentinels when they pose a risk of zoonotic transmission or when they serve as a reservoir species for the pathogen. Even so, companion animals remain valuable incidental sentinels.

Cat scratch disease

Since the identification of *Bartonella henselae*, the etiologic agent of cat scratch disease (CSD), in the early 1990s, cats have served as the only population for CSD surveillance, primarily through serosurveillance. Recent studies have indicated that dogs can be naturally infected with at least six species of *Bartonella*, including *B henselae*, and may also function as sentinels, as all *Bartonella* spp identified in sick dogs are also pathogenic or potentially pathogenic in humans. Unlike cats, which rarely exhibit clinical disease following bartonella infection, dogs develop a wide range of clinical abnormalities very similar to those observed following bartonella infection in people. For example, infection with *B vinsonii* subspecies *berkhoffii*, produces endocarditis with similar lesions in both dogs and people.[14] Due to similarities between clinical signs in canine and human bartonella spp infection, the canine species may be a good sentinel species for CSD and other potential bartonella infections of humans.[14,15] One caveat is the potential risk of transmission between infected dogs and people.

Rocky Mountain spotted fever

The spotted fever group diseases represent over a dozen species of *Rickettsia*, several of which have importance as globally re-emerging diseases. Rocky Mountain spotted fever, caused by *Rickettsia rickettsii,* is an important tick-borne disease of both dogs and people in North, Central, and South America. Reports in North and

South America have demonstrated parallels in human and canine infection within households and across geographic areas.[16-18] Close contact between dogs and tick habitats makes them a sensitive indicator of the environmental presence of infected vectors and useful as sentinels for other household members or others in the same geographic location. Because dogs infected with Rocky Mountain spotted fever do not present a direct transmission risk to people, they have potential usefulness as both intentional and incidental animal sentinels, although theoretically they could transfer infected ticks to the peridomestic environment.

Leishmaniasis

Leishmaniasis, a vector-borne disease of worldwide concern, is transmitted by the bite of infected female phlebotamine sandflies and manifests as either a cutaneous or visceral form. The World Health Organization indicates that nearly 350 million people are at risk of leishmaniasis in 88 countries around the world.[19] While most human cases of leishmaniasis in the United States can be traced to exposures outside North America, a few cases of domestically acquired cutaneous leishmaniasis have been reported in Texas.[20] Companion animals, including dogs, cats, and horses, are also susceptible to leishmaniasis.[21] In endemic regions of Columbia and Panama, dogs have been used as sentinels for detection of leishmania spp transmission.[22,23] For nonendemic regions, clinical diagnosis of canine leishmaniasis or evidence of seroconversion to *Leishmania* spp may indicate an isolated imported case or expansion of endemic regions due to an extended vector range or introduction of the parasite into a new vector or reservoir species. Evidence of an outbreak of canine visceral leishmaniasis in a New York kennel in 1999 prompted an investigation of the epidemiology of *Leishmania* spp in North America. While no evidence of human infection was found in the 3-year study, infected dogs were identified in 18 states and two Canadian provinces. Evidence of newly infected dogs during each year of the study indicated the occurrence of ongoing disease transmission.[24] Clear evidence of clinical illness or seroconversion in infected dogs, their potential for exposure to the sandfly vector, and the absence of direct transmission from dogs to humans are desirable sentinel characteristics in dogs. However, dogs can serve as a reservoir for *Leishmania* spp, which limits their use as intentional sentinels for disease surveillance.

Trypanosomiasis

Trypanosoma cruzi represents another important public health concern where companion animals may be effectively used as sentinels across the American continents. American trypanosomiasis, or Chagas disease, is a vector-borne disease transmitted during the simultaneous feeding and defecation on hosts by blood-sucking members of the family Reduviidae. Chagas disease affects many animal species, including cats, dogs, mice, and rats. Most human cases of Chagas disease in North America are traced to exposure in endemic regions of Mexico, Central America, and South America, but cases of transmission in the United States have also been documented.[25] *T cruzi* is considered to be endemic in eastern, southern, and southwestern regions of the United States with opossums and raccoons serving as natural reservoirs.[26] Serologic evidence of exposure to *T cruzi* has been found in hounds from the southeastern and central United States as well as the Canadian province of Ontario.[24] As with leishmaniasis, dogs can exhibit clinical or serologic signs of trypanosoma cruzi infection without the risk of direct disease transmission to humans. Therefore, dogs may serve as valuable sentinels for Chagas disease in nonendemic areas to monitor geographic spread of the disease as well as the effectiveness of vector control programs and other preventive measures.[27] However, as a main reservoir species for *T cruzi* in endemic regions, dogs may be limited for service only as incidental sentinels for disease surveillance.

Environmental Contaminants

While companion animals share the same air, water, and housing as their owners, they tend to be free of many lifestyle factors that can confound associations with true risk factors. Lifestyle factors often associated with chronic disease in people include tobacco use, alcohol and caffeine consumption, poor diet, insufficient physical inactivity, and low social class. The physiologically compressed life span of companion animals also makes them valuable sentinels for many diseases where lengthy latency periods associated with the human life span preclude early detection of many hazardous environmental conditions.

Lead poisoning

Lead exposure in people and animals has well-known and well-documented detrimental clinical effects. Identical biological mechanisms of toxicity in both people and animals, including companion animals, have allowed for the successful use of dogs as animal models for toxicologic studies of lead exposure.[28–30] The use of companion animals as sentinels for environmental lead contamination has also been successful in determining human health risk for plumbism. For example, both dogs and cats suffering from plumbism have led to the discovery and successful treatment of nonclinical lead toxicity in children living in the same household.[31]

Environmental lead exposure beyond the household environment can also be determined through serologic surveillance of blood-lead concentrations in both cats and dogs. A study of pets and their owners living near a secondary lead smelter in Illinois found that when a dog or cat in a household had a high blood-lead concentration, there was a significant increase in the likelihood of finding a person in the same household with a high blood-lead concentration.[32] In Uruguay, similar findings were reported following investigation of the "La Teja" neighborhood, where people settled into an area of abandoned lead-handling factories. While blood-lead concentrations were significantly higher in dogs than in children, correlation between high blood-lead concentrations in dogs and children was evident.[33]

While both dogs and cats share similar household environmental exposures with their owners, dogs exhibit behavioral traits more in common with children. Like children, dogs explore the environment low to the ground and may eat or chew objects they discover. These behavior similarities between dogs and children make dogs the better choice for incidental animal-sentinel surveillance related to lead exposure.

Organochlorines

Dioxins, a group of several hundred similar chemical compounds, have been linked to increased risk of cancer development, adverse reproductive effects, and developmental abnormalities in both people and animals.[34–36] While wildlife species have been key animal sentinels for determining the environmental risk of dioxins for human and animal health,[11] the use of companion animals as sentinels for environmental dioxins is not as well defined. In an investigation of the health effects of 2,3,7,8:tetrachlorodibenzodioxin (TCDD), the most toxic of the dioxin compounds, on pets in Missouri, researchers were unable to confirm the usefulness of either cats or dogs as potential animal sentinels. However, researchers relied on owner-reported illness to determine if pets were likely suffering from TCDD toxicity. TCDD exposure was assumed based on owner's exposure risk rather than serum or tissue testing. Along with small sample size and lack of typical reported signs of toxicity, the investigators reported their results as inconclusive.[37] Conversely, a study of environmental exposure of dogs to PCB, another common dioxin compound, found them to be a potentially useful animal sentinel for environmental PCB exposure. In this study, serum PCB levels in dogs from known areas of contamination in Monroe County, Indiana, were significantly higher than levels in control dogs from noncontaminated areas in Atlanta, Georgia. Interestingly there was no association between being an outdoor dog and having higher serum PCB levels, as would be expected if soil exposure to PCBs significantly contributed to exposure.[38] Unfortunately neither the PCB nor the TCDD studies were able to correlate outcomes in companion animals with their owners, as outcomes in the owners were not measured. Until those studies are completed, the usefulness of companion animals as sentinels for environmental dioxin risk in people will remain inconclusive.

Organochlorine pesticides such as DDT, its active metabolite DDE (dichlorodiphenyldichloroethylene), and lindane have also been implicated in numerous health risks ranging from neurologic symptoms to adverse reproductive effects to cancer development.[39] Dogs living near Superfund sites in North Carolina had a significantly higher micronucleus frequency, a biomarker for DNA damage, than did dogs from nearby noncontaminated areas. While not all measured biomarkers differed between the exposed and control dogs, this study suggests that dogs may be useful sentinels when carefully chosen biomarkers are used.[40] However, as with the dioxins, correlations between human and animal health risk have not been determined for the organochlorine pesticides, and extrapolations based on available data should be done with caution.

Industrial chemicals

Between May 1 and August 31, 2006, a community in Georgia was exposed to propyl mercaptan, an offensive smelling chemical used to scent odorless toxic chemicals, following the accidental release of propyl mercaptan from a nonhazardous waste-treatment facility. During the initial investigation, a community survey was conducted that included a section for owner-reported signs of illness in pets. Follow-up on the 36 pets with reported illnesses determined that only 6 animals were seen by a veterinarian. Of the 8 sick pets reported to have died during the study period, only 1 had a necropsy performed, with findings consistent with gastric torsion.[41] The lack of veterinary confirmation of disease and cause of death and reliance on owner-reported clinical signs made it difficult to evaluate dogs as sentinels for environmental contamination of propyl mercaptan during this event. Using data from veterinary hospitals, the National Companion Animal Surveillance Program conducted a second study on pets as sentinels during the same event. This retrospective syndromic surveillance study found indications of changes in respiratory, gastrointestinal, and eye inflammation syndromes concurrent with the chemical exposure. These syndromes paralleled reports of clinical complaints by people in the affected community, but showed no conclusive and consistent evidence of adverse health effects.[42] The results of this study support the need for further studies on the use of companion animals as sentinels following chemical accidents and for the development and evaluation of methods for using pet medical records for the detection of environmental health hazards.

Bioterrorism and Chemical Terrorism

Since the terrorist attacks on September 11, 2001, there is an increased awareness of potential biological, chemical and radiological threats, which has led to increased efforts for early detection of terrorist attacks. Animal-sentinel surveillance has been proposed as an early detection warning system for terrorist attacks.[43,44] If companion-animal species develop rapid clinical signs of illness, identification of an attack can be made before detection of disease in people. This rapid detection may allow for early interventions designed to decrease the impact of the attack on both animal and human health.

The CDC has categorized biological agents into three categories, depending on how easily they can be spread, the severity of illness they might cause, and the likelihood of deaths that might result. Category A agents are considered the highest risk and category C agents are those that are considered emerging threats for disease.[45] Listed biological agents that can cause clinical disease in companion animals include anthrax, brucellosis, plague, and tularemia. Vector-borne diseases, such as some species of *Rickettsia,* may also have potential as effective bioterrorism agents.[46] In addition, numerous chemical agents have been identified as potential terrorist weapons. Neurologic gases, heavy metals (eg, mercury and lead), cyanide compounds, pesticides, dioxin, and PCBs are all identified by the CDC as chemical agents that may be used by terrorists.[45]

A single case of lead toxicity in a dog or tularemia in two cats from the same household are not likely to lead a veterinarian to suspect bioterrorism. However, a veterinarian is in a good position to see larger trends that might be a tip off of a terrorist attack. By tracking the incidence of disease in an individual practice, a veterinarian can recognize unusual increases in the incidence of specific disease or disease syndromes. Companion animals also have the potential to become sensitive animal sentinels for bioterrorism or chemical terrorism attacks as a part of a larger syndromic surveillance system.

SUMMARY

Animal-sentinel surveillance is a key component of public health risk assessment. To be effective sentinels, animals must be susceptible to the disease of interest and create a measurable response to the disease. Ideally, animal sentinels do not pose a threat of direct disease transmission to people or serve as an amplifying host or reservoir for the disease. While many species serve as animal sentinels, companion animals have an especially valuable role as sentinels because of their unique place in people's lives, with exposure to similar household and recreational risk factors as those for the people who own them. Incidents of food contamination, infectious disease, environmental contamination, and even bioterrorism or chemical terrorism events may be detected in dogs and cats before disease is detected in people. In any of these events, communication between veterinarians and public health officials can facilitate rapid detection of disease and implementation of disease-control and -prevention strategies to ultimately minimize detrimental health effects in both people and animals.

REFERENCES

1. Kuchta D. Mine canaries. Anthracite History Journal. Available at: http://www.minecountry.com/homeMine/dispart.cfm?id=15. Accessed July 21, 2008.
2. McClusky B. Use of sentinel herds in monitoring and surveillance systems. In: Salman MD, editor. Animal disease surveillance and survey systems. Ames (IA): Iowa State Press; 2003. p. 119–33.
3. Halliday JEB, Meredith AL, Knobel DL, et al. A framework for evaluating animals as sentinels for infectious disease surveillance. J R Soc Interface 2007;4(16): 973–84.
4. Cano JP, Dee SA, Murtaugh MP, et al. Impact of a modified-live porcine reproductive and respiratory syndrome virus vaccine intervention on a population of pigs infected with a heterologous isolate. Am J Vet Res 2007;68(5):565–71.

5. Gillespie TG, Carroll AL. Methods of control and elimination of porcine reproductive and respiratory syndrome virus using modified live virus vaccine in a two-site production system. J Swine Health Prod 2003;11(6):291–5.

6. Pfeiffer DU, Minh PQ, Martin V, et al. An analysis of the spatial and temporal patterns of highly pathogenic avian influenza occurrence in Vietnam using national surveillance data. Vet J 2007;174(2):302–9.

7. Mannelli A, Busani L, Toson M, et al. Transmission parameters of highly pathogenic avian influenza (H7N1) among industrial poultry farms in northern Italy in 1999–2000. Prev Vet Med 2007;81(4):318–22.

8. Senne DA. Avian influenza in North and South America, 2002–2005. Avian Dis 2007;51(Suppl 1):167–73.

9. Krauss S, Obert CA, Franks, et al. Influenza in migratory birds and evidence of limited intercontinental virus exchange. PLoS Pathog 2007;3(11):1684–93.

10. Cardona CJ, Xing Z, Sandrock CE, et al. Avian influenza in birds and animals. Comp Immunol Microbiol Infect Dis; 10.1016/j.cimid.2008.01.001, in press.

11. Fox GA. Wildlife as sentinels of human health effects in the Great Lakes–St. Lawrence basin. Environ Health Perspect 2001;109(Suppl 6):853–61.

12. Burns K. Chief executive officers testify about recall of pet food. J Am Vet Med Assoc 2007;230(11):1600–2.

13. Burns K. Hogs, chickens at pet food containing adulterants. J Am Vet Med Assoc 2007;230(11):1603.

14. Chomel BB, Boulouis HJ, Maruyama S, et al. *Bartonella* spp. in pets and effect on human health. Emerg Infect Dis 2006;12(3):389–94.

15. Henn JB, Gabriel MW, Kasten RW, et al. Gray foxes (Urocyon cinereoargenteus) as a potential reservoir of a Bartonella clarridgeiae-like bacterium and domestic dogs as part of a sentinel system for surveillance of zoonotic arthropod-borne pathogens in northern California. J Clin Microbiol 2007;45(8):2411–8.

16. Elchos BN, Goddard J. Implications of presumptive fatal Rocky mountain spotted fever in two dogs and their owner. J Am Vet Med Assoc 2003;223(10):1450–2.

17. Kidd L, Hegarty B, Sexton D, et al. Molecular characterization of *Rickettsia rickettsii* infecting dogs and people in North Carolina. Ann N Y Acad Sci 2006;1078:400–9.

18. Pinter A, Horta MC, Pacheco RC, et al. Serosurvey of *Rickettsia* spp. in dogs and humans from an endemic area for Brazilian spotted fever in the state of São Paulo. Brazil. Cad. Saúde Pública 2008;24(2):247–52.

19. World Health Organization. Leishmaniasis: the disease and its epidemiology. Available at: http://www.who.int/leishmaniasis/disease_epidemiology/en/index.html. Accessed July 24, 2008.

20. Centers for Disease Control and Prevention. Division of parasitic diseases. Fact sheet: leishmania infection. Available at: http://www.cdc.gov/ncidod/dpd/parasites/leishmania/factsht_leishmania.htm. Accessed July 24, 2008.

21. Gramiccia M, Gradoni L. The current status of zoonotic leishmaniasis and approaches to disease control. Int J Parasitol 2005;35(11–12):1169–80.

22. Corredor A, Gallego JF, Tesh RB, et al. Epidemiology of visceral leishmaniasis in Colombia. Am J Trop Med Hyg 1989;40(5):480–6.

23. Herrer A, Christensen HA, Beumer RJ. Detection of leishmanial activity in nature by means of sentinel animals. Trans R Soc Trop Med Hyg 1973;67(6):870–9.

24. Duprey ZH, Steurer FJ, Rooney JA, et al. Canine visceral leishmaniasis, United States and Canada, 2000–2003. Emerg Infect Dis 2006;12(3):440–6.

25. Centers for Disease Control and Prevention. Chagas disease: epidemiology and risk factors. Available at: http://www.cdc.gov/chagas/epi.html. Accessed July 24, 2008.

26. Roellig DM, Brown EL, Barnabé C, et al. Molecular typing of Trypanosoma cruzi isolates, United States. Emerg Infect Dis 2008;14(7):1123–5.

27. Castañera MB, Lauricella MA, Chuit R, et al. Evaluation of dogs as sentinels of the transmission of Trypanosoma cruzi in a rural area of north-western Argentina. Ann Trop Med Parasitol 1998;92(6):671–83.

28. Stowe HD, Goyer RA, Krigman M, et al. Experimental oral lead toxicity in young dogs. Clinical and morphologic effects. Arch Pathol 1973;95(2):106–16.

29. Caldwell KC, Taddeini L, Woodburn RL, et al. Induction of myeloperoxidase deficiency in granulocytes in lead-intoxicated dogs. Blood 1979;53(4):588–93.

30. Stowe HD, Vandevelde M. Lead-induced encephalopathy in dogs fed high fat, low calcium diets. J Neuropathol Exp Neurol 1979;38(5):463–74.

31. Dowsett R, Shannon M. Childhood plumbism identified after lead poisoning in household pets. N Engl J Med 1994;331(24):1661–2.

32. Berny PJ, Côté LM, Buck WB. Can household pets be used as reliable monitors of lead exposure to humans? Sci Total Environ 1995;172(2–3):163–73.

33. Mañay N, Cousillas AZ, Alvarez C, et al. Lead contamination in Uruguay: the "La Teja" neighborhood case. Rev Environ Contam Toxicol 2008;195:93–115.

34. Cole P, Trichopoulos D, Pastides H, et al. Dioxin and cancer: a critical review. Regul Toxicol Pharmacol 2003;38(3):378–88.

35. Arisawa K, Takeda H, Mikasa H. Background exposure to PCDDs/PCDFs/PCBs and its potential health effects: a review of epidemiologic studies. J Med Invest 2005;52(1–2):10–21.

36. Carpenter DO. Polychlorinated biphenyls (PCBs): routes of exposure and effects on human health. Rev Environ Health 2006;21(1):1–23.

37. Schilling RJ, Stehr-Green PA. Health effects in family pets and 2,3,7,8-TCDD contamination in Missouri: a look at potential animal sentinels. Arch Environ Health 1987;42(3):137–9.

38. Schilling RJ, Steele GK, Harris AE, et al. Canine serum levels of polychlorinated biphenyls (PCBs): a pilot study to evaluate the use of animal sentinels in environmental health. Arch Environ Health 1988;43(3):218–21.

39. Rogan WJ, Chen A. Health risks and benefits of bis(4-chlorophenyl)-1,1, 1-trichloroethane (DDT). Lancet 2005;366(9487):763–73.

40. Backer LC, Grindem CB, Corbett WT, et al. Pet dogs as sentinels for environmental contamination. Sci Total Environ 2001;274(1–3):161–9.

41. Gdhr-Dph, Atsdr. Health consultation: PSC recovery systems fairburn, Fullerton County, Georgia. Available at: http://www.atsdr.cdc.gov/HAC/pha/PSC_Recovery_Systems/PSCRecoverySystems030708.pdf. March 7, 2008. Accessed July 24, 2008.

42. Maciejewski R, Glickman N, Moore G, et al. Companion animals as sentinels for community exposure to industrial chemicals: the Fairburn, GA, propyl mercaptan case study. Public Health Rep 2008;123(3):333–42.

43. Rabinowitz P, Gordon Z, Chudnov D, et al. Animals as sentinels of bioterrorism agents. Emerg Infect Dis 2006;12(4):647–52.

44. Rabinowitz P, Wiley J, Odofin L, et al. Animals as sentinels of chemical terrorism agents: an evidence-based review. Clin Toxicol (Phila) 2008;46(2):93–100.

45. Anonymous. Biological and chemical terrorism: strategic plan for preparedness and response. MMWR Recomm Rep 2000;49(RR-4):1–14.

46. Azad AF, Radulovic S. Pathogenic rickettsiae as bioterrorism agents. Ann N Y Acad Sci 2003;990:734–8.

Influenza in Dogs and Cats

Emily Beeler, DVM[a,b,*]

KEYWORDS

- Influenza • Dog • Cat • Emerging disease • H5N1 • H3N8

For the first time in history, influenza viruses have been documented as the cause of natural outbreaks of illness in dogs and cats. The years 2003 to 2004 brought the discovery of both canine influenza (H3N8) in racing greyhounds in Florida and avian influenza (H5N1) in zoo cats in Thailand. Dogs and cats may come to play a role in the evolution of new strains of human influenza. As a result, small animal veterinarians face new challenges in caring for their patients and a heightened public health responsibility. Canine influenza (H3N8), which is not known to be zoonotic, is the strain small animal practitioners are most likely to encounter. However, veterinarians must also be aware of less common, but perhaps more consequential, strains.

INFLUENZA BASICS

Influenza viruses belong to the family Orthomyxoviridae. There are three major types of influenza: A, B, and C.[1] Influenza A, which is the focus of this article, is of the greatest significance: it is the most mutable, causes human influenza pandemics, and has the widest host species range.[2]

Influenza A is an enveloped virus. The envelope, derived from the plasma membrane of the cell in which the virus was assembled, makes influenza A easier to inactivate than nonenveloped viruses.[3] Cold temperatures prolong survival of influenza virus in water and on surfaces. It is inactivated by most properly performed cleaning and disinfection protocols. Heat, common disinfectants, hand washing, and laundering are all useful in reducing contamination (**Table 1**).

The influenza A genome contains eight separate strands of RNA that code for 11 proteins. Two of the 11 are called hemagglutinin (H) and neuraminidase (N).[4]

[a] Los Angeles County Department of Public Health, Veterinary Public Health and Rabies Control Program, 7601 East Imperial Highway, Building 700, Room 94A, Downey, CA 90242, USA
[b] College of Veterinary Medicine, Western University of Health Sciences, 309 E Second Street, Pomona, CA 91766, USA
* Los Angeles County Department of Public Health, Veterinary Public Health and Rabies Control Program, 7601 E Imperial Highway, Building 700, Room 94A, Downey, CA 90242, USA.
E-mail address: ebeeler@ph.lacounty.gov

Vet Clin Small Anim 39 (2009) 251–264
doi:10.1016/j.cvsm.2008.10.011
0195-5616/08/$ – see front matter © 2009 Elsevier Inc. All rights reserved.

Table 1
Influenza A survival times, inactivation periods, and inactivation procedures for various environmental conditions

Environment	Survival Time for Influenza A Viruses
Water	
Frozen	Indefinitely
32°F	Over 30 days
71°F	4 days
132°F–140°F	0.5–3 hours[45]
Feces (generally from infected birds)	
Frozen	Indefinitely
39°F	30–35 days
68°F	7 days[45]
Cloth, paper, tissues (no visible organic matter)	8–12 hours[46]
Nonporous plastic, stainless steel (with no visible organic matter)	1–2 days[46]

Sanitation Need	Procedure
Hand cleaning	Warm soap and water for ≥20 seconds. If no organic matter is adhered to hands, alcohol-based hand sanitizer may be used; enough should be applied to keep hands moist for ≥20 seconds.[47]
Surface disinfection (after visible organic matter removed)	1% bleach, 70% ethanol, quaternary ammonium salts (such as Roccal or Triple 2), and many other disinfectants. Contact time ≥10 minutes.[48]
Towels, bedding, cloth	Normal laundering with detergent[47]
Instrument sterilization	Moist heat autoclaving at 250°F for 15 minutes, at 140°F for 30 minutes,[48] or cold sterilization with glutaraldehyde solutions.[43]
Cooking	Heat to minimum of 165°F[49]

Numerous copies of these two proteins project through the envelope and appear as "spikes" coating the viral surface (**Fig. 1**).

Hemagglutinins allow the virus to attach to sialic acid receptors on cell surfaces and thereby infect cells. Hemagglutinin plays the predominant role in the species specificity and tissue tropism of the virus. Sixteen different serotypes of hemagglutinin have been identified: H1 to H16.[5]

Neuraminidase orchestrates the exit of newly formed virons from an infected cell by cleaving sialic acid receptors that would otherwise bind to the hemagglutinin. Nine neuraminidase serotypes have been discovered.[1] Influenza A viruses are subcategorized by these two surface proteins. Examples include H1N1, H5N1, and H9N2.

MUTATION

The mutability of influenza A leads to annual outbreaks of influenza and occasional pandemics. Mutation occurs two ways.

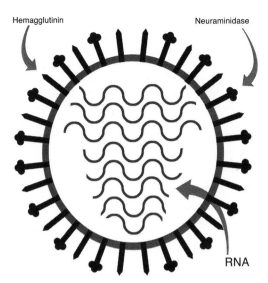

Fig. 1. Hemagglutinin and neuraminidase surface proteins, influenza A virus.

In antigenic "drift," single nucleic acid point mutations occur when influenza RNA is replicated within an infected cell. There is no "proofreader" enzyme to correct these mutations. Drift causes the constant low-level change seen in human seasonal flu.

In antigenic "shift" the host range of an influenza virus abruptly changes. Typically two different influenza viruses enter the same cell and swap genes during replication. These new viruses may have a different host range than the original viruses.[5]

ECOLOGY OF INFLUENZA A VIRUSES

Wild waterfowl are the reservoir for all known influenza A subtypes.[1] Many influenza A viruses replicate in the birds' intestinal mucosa and are shed in feces, without causing apparent illness. Periodically, new influenza A strains emerge from the wild, adapt to new species, and cause epizootics or panzootics.[1]

Most of the time, however, influenza viruses exhibit species-specific infectivity. An individual strain of influenza is highly contagious, or highly adapted, to only one species (**Table 2**). The most common strains of influenza A infect humans, poultry, pigs, horses, and dogs.[2] Outbreaks have been documented in harbor seals.[6] Ferrets are susceptible to human influenza viruses.[2] The H5N1 avian influenza virus is

Table 2		
Adaptedness of influenza A strains infecting humans, cats and dogs		
Species	**Well Adapted:** **Highly Transmissible Between** **Members of Same Species**	**Partly Adapted:** **Not Highly Transmissible Between** **Members of Same Species**
Humans	H3N2, H1N1	H5N1, H9N2, H7N2, H7N3, H7N7[5]
Cats	None known.	H5N1[19–30]
Dogs	H3N8[39–43]	H5N1, H3N2[11,34–38]

transmissible between cats on a small scale, but has not been shown to spread rapidly or efficiently in cats.

A large number of influenza A viruses infect poultry. Clinical signs are primarily seen in chickens and turkeys, and ducks are often asymptomatic. Virus is shed in feces and respiratory secretions. Most avian influenza viruses are considered low pathogenicity avian influenza (LPAI) viruses, causing drops in egg production and mild respiratory signs. A subset of LPAI viruses, those containing hemagglutinins H7 or H5, can mutate to become highly pathogenic avian influenza (HPAI) viruses. HPAI causes sudden death, dyspnea, diarrhea, cyanosis, neurologic signs, and hemorrhage and necrosis in multiple internal organs.[7]

PANDEMIC INFLUENZA

The influenza pandemic of 1918 to 1919 was one of the largest and most severe human disease outbreaks in history, taking up to 50 million lives.[5] This virus was later labeled an H1N1 influenza A virus. Half of the deaths were in healthy adults. Many died from acute respiratory distress syndrome (ARDS).[8]

Genetic sequencing of the 1918 virus suggests it originated when a bird strain transferred to and adapted to humans; it was an entirely new virus in the human population, unrelated to the seasonal influenza of the time. The originating bird host remains a mystery. In contrast, milder human influenza pandemics in 1957 and 1968 followed mutation of the circulating seasonal influenza virus, which had acquired a few genes from avian viruses.[9]

CONCERNS FOR A NEW PANDEMIC

It is unknown if new pandemics can be predicted.[8] In recent years, five influenza A subtypes of avian origin have been transmitted to humans, causing illness without becoming highly transmissible from human to human (see **Table 2**). All are candidates for becoming the next pandemic strain. One of them, HPAI H5N1, has spread over a vast geographic area and caused the greatest concern.

HIGHLY PATHOGENIC AVIAN INFLUENZA H5N1

HPAI H5N1 is causing one of the largest panzootics in poultry ever documented, and has crossed the species barrier several times, infecting humans, tigers, leopards, domestic cats, palm civets (a kind of exotic cat), macaques, a stone marten (a weasel-like animal), a mink, and a few dogs.[10–12] It first caused poultry outbreaks in Hong Kong in 1997 and later spread throughout Southeast Asia, westward across Asia, and into Europe, the Middle East, and Africa. Wild waterfowl, the typically asymptomatic reservoirs of influenza A, died from HPAI H5N1 by the thousands in 2005 and 2006 at a large lake in China.[10]

Human infections with HPAI H5N1 are infrequent, occurring in places where poultry outbreaks occur, with a case fatality rate of 60%. Most people are infected by very close contact with infected poultry or their feces, or ingestion of raw poultry products.[10] There are isolated cases of human-to-human transmission of the virus. Infected humans exhibit respiratory signs and fever, with many developing ARDS. Neurologic signs and diarrhea can also occur. Elevated aspartate aminotransferase (AST), alanine transaminase (ALT), and creatinine have been found in some patients. Lymphopenia upon presentation is statistically associated with a higher case fatality rate.[13] The HPAI H5N1 virus attaches best to human bronchiolar epithelium and alveoli, and poorly to the tracheal epithelium. Preferential binding occurs to Type II pneumocytes, which produce surfactant and are more metabolically active than Type I cells. Perhaps the most telling, H5N1 adheres very well to pulmonary macrophages, which plays a role in inflammation and ARDS.[14,15]

There have been few autopsies performed in cases of human HPAI H5N1. Feline cases, although less closely reported and tracked, have been documented in much greater detail.

INFLUENZA IN CATS

Experiments in the 1970s and 1980s showed that cats could become infected with human influenza A (H3N2, H2N2). They shed the virus from the nose or pharynx, developed an antibody response, and transmitted it from cat-to-cat, but did not become ill.[15–17] Before the appearance of HPAI H5N1, there were no known natural occurrences of influenza A illness in cats.

HIGHLY PATHOGENIC AVIAN INFLUENZA H5N1 IN CATS

In February 2004, the World Health Organization reported a die-off of 14 out of 15 cats in one household in Thailand. Two of three cats tested were positive for H5N1. At least one of these cats had been in contact with dead chickens.[18]

Subsequent reports identified H5N1 infection in tigers in China,[19] tigers and leopards from zoos in Thailand,[20,21] a domestic cat in Thailand,[22] domestic cats in Iraq and Turkey,[23] three stray cats on a German island,[24] and cats in an Austrian animal shelter.[25] In all cases, except that in the Austrian shelter, cats were found dead or had severe illness. Clinical signs included high fever, dyspnea, panting, ataxia, and convulsions. In most of these cases, ingestion of raw infected birds or direct contact with poultry feces were likely sources. A serosurvey of stray cats near infected poultry markets showed that 20% were seropositive, indicating prior infection.[26] There have been no reports of humans contracting the virus from cats.

The 2004 outbreak of H5N1 in a tiger zoo in Thailand happened after tigers ate raw, infected chickens. The cats' diet was changed to cooked meat and moribund cats were euthanized to stop the outbreak. More cats became ill despite the intervention, and tiger-to-tiger transmission was suspected.[21]

The 2006 report of H5N1 infection in three cats in an Austrian animal shelter was not associated with clinical signs. Cats had been tested because some had climbed into a poultry pen where an H5N1-infected swan was kept. Only 3 of 40 cats tested were positive for viral RNA on pharyngeal swabs. A week later two of these cats were rechecked, and were negative. These two cats did seroconvert, as did another cat that had been negative for viral RNA on pharyngeal swab.[25] Some feared this meant cats could silently carry and shed the virus. However, given the very limited spread of the virus under shelter conditions, this is unlikely to be the case. It is not known if any cats had shed live virus.

Results of experimental studies on HPAI H5N1 infection in cats are similar to what has been observed in the field. Cats inoculated oculo-nasopharyngeally, intratracheally, or by being fed infected 1-day old chicks, developed high fevers (over 104°F), dyspnea, conjunctivitis, and prominent nictitans. Infected cats transmitted the virus to their uninfected cage mates. These secondarily infected cats also became very ill. Clinical signs began 1 to 2 days postinfection for those experimentally infected and about 5 days after exposure to ill cats for those infected secondarily. Cats did *not* become infected when living next to or sharing bowls with infected dogs, nor did infected cats transmit virus to dogs. Swabs taken of the pharynx and rectum of ill cats revealed viral RNA, raising the possibility that virus might be shed in feces and possibly be spread through the fecal-oral route. Feces from the cats were not reported to be evaluated directly for virus.[27-30]

Necropsies from both the naturally occurring and experimentally infected cases revealed systemic pathology, similar to that seen in chickens infected with HPAI H5N1. Commonly seen were hemorrhagic consolidated lungs, and bronchointerstitial and necrotic pneumonia with loss of bronchiolar and alveolar epithelium. Liver necrosis and encephalitis were also frequent. In some cases, enlarged tonsils and mandibular lymph nodes, pleural effusion, hemorrhagic pancreatitis, and hemorrhage in multiple organs was seen. Virus was found in the lungs, liver, and brain by immunohistochemistry and virus isolation.[20-24,27-30] Virus was also extracted from pleural fluid, duodenum, kidney, spleen, and urine of the infected domestic cat from Thailand.[22]

A dose-response in cat H5N1 infections has been demonstrated. When inoculated with high doses of virus, cats become severely ill as seen before. When inoculated with moderate doses, cats showed no clinical signs, but seroconverted and shed some virus from the pharynx. Cats inoculated with small amounts of virus do not become ill, seroconvert, or shed any virus.[30]

Cats were protected from HPAI H5N1 by an experimental vaccine created from an LPAI H5N6 virus. The vaccine was administered to five cats subcutaneously, twice to each cat, 1 month apart. A month after the second dose, they were challenged with high doses of HPAI H5N1 virus. They developed only mild fevers, with the highest being 102.7°F, and no other clinical signs. In contrast, unvaccinated control cats became severely ill. Only two of the five vaccinated cats shed any viral RNA from the pharynx and rectum after H5N1 inoculation, and only one shed live virus. This last cat had produced the lowest levels of H5N1-specific antibodies in response to the vaccine. In contrast, all five cats used as unvaccinated controls shed large amounts of virus from the pharynx after infection, and two shed virus rectally.[30] The successful use of an imperfectly matched vaccine to protect cats and reduce viral shedding is encouraging for future efforts to protect both human and feline health.

The issue of cat-to-cat spread has triggered a great deal of concern. If the virus were to circulate more extensively in cats, it might adapt better to both humans and cats. H5N1 virus binds preferentially deep in the lungs in cats just as it does in humans[14] and causes ARDS-like illness. The virus is shed rectally in both species.[10,28] Because the behavior of the virus in cats and humans is so similar, it could theoretically be transmitted between these two species.

COMMUNICATING WITH THE PUBLIC, CALMING FEARS

Many pet owners became fearful following instances of cats infected with HPAI H5N1.[31] Animal shelters in Germany reported a surge of phone calls and an increase in people seeking to relinquish their pets. Authorities feared a wave of cat-killings and clarified that it was illegal to shoot strays.[31] The provision of clear advice from European authorities for regions that had had H5N1-positive birds helped to minimize public anxiety (**Box 1**).There have been no reports of cats infected with H5N1 in Europe since 2006, despite continued detection of the virus in European wild birds and poultry. The precautions recommended by the European Centers for Disease Control and Prevention appear to have been effective. There have been no reported human cases of H5N1 in Europe.

Dr Albert Osterhaus, a veterinarian researching influenza in cats, pointed out that H5N1-infected cats excrete 0.1% or less of the amount of virus that chickens do.[32] Should HPAI H5N1 mutate, adapt fully to humans, and cause the next human pandemic, then contagion from infected humans, not cats, would be the main concern.

30 days, and nasal discharge that may be either serous or purulent. A subset of dogs develop high fever (104°F to 106°F) and pneumonia. The case fatality rate is between 1% and 5%.[44]

Diagnosis

Canine influenza H3N8 should be suspected in outbreaks of respiratory disease among fully vaccinated dogs. Serology is one of the most useful diagnostic approaches. Infected dogs typically seroconvert by day 7 after the onset of clinical signs. In locations where canine influenza is not yet endemic, a single positive serum antibody titer combined with compatible symptoms is suggestive of the disease. A fourfold increase in titer 2 to 3 weeks later confirms it. Serum samples may be shipped on ice packs directly to the Cornell Animal Health Diagnostic Center for testing. For details, see: http://diaglab.vet.cornell.edu/issues/civ.asp#samp.

Polymerase chain reaction (PCR)-based testing for the RNA of the virus may be performed on nasal swabs. They are most accurate if samples are collected from infected dogs before clinical signs appear.[44] A negative result does not rule out infection. Viral shedding begins before the onset of clinical signs and tapers throughout the first 2 to 3 days of illness. Many dogs are likely to no longer be shedding by the time they present to a veterinarian. Lung and distal trachea can be tested by PCR in fatal cases. The Cornell Animal Health Diagnostic Center and the University of California at Davis, Lucy Whittier Molecular and Diagnostic Core Facility, offer PCR testing for the virus. For details, see the above link for Cornell or the following for UC Davis: http://www.vetmed.ucdavis.edu/vme/taqmanservice/pdfs/DiagnosticPacket.pdf.

Treatment and Control

Educating staff and dog owners about protocols for preventing contagion should be an integral part of treatment, whether the dog is hospitalized or treated at home.

The virus is easily transmitted through direct contact between dogs and through aerosolization (ie, coughing and sneezing). Humans may play a role in fomite transmission by touching an infected dog, then touching surfaces that other dog handlers come in contact with, such as doorknobs. Staff should change their clothes before going home to prevent bringing the virus home to their own dogs.[44]

Suspect cases entering the clinic should be escorted to an examination room immediately. The floors, walls, and tables of the room should be thoroughly disinfected after use, with special attention to doorknobs and other objects that humans may touch. To prevent further transmission, dog owners should be counseled to isolate cases at home until recovery, to wash hands and food bowls and water bowls frequently with soap, and to change clothes before handling other dogs.

Hospitalized cases should be placed in isolation. At minimum, gloves and gown should be worn while handling the canine influenza patient. Hands should be washed with soap and water or disinfected with alcohol-based hand sanitizer after handling the dog. Shoes should be disinfected with an appropriately maintained disinfectant footbath upon exiting isolation. As with all influenza viruses, thorough cleaning and disinfection procedures inactivate the virus (see **Table 1**).[40]

There is no recommended specific treatment for canine influenza,[40,44] but broad-spectrum antibiotics are often used to control secondary bacterial infection and may reduce purulent nasal discharge. For pneumonia cases, transtracheal wash and culture may be needed to identify secondary bacterial infections.[44] Supportive treatment includes intravenous fluids, bronchodilators, coupage, and supplemental oxygen. Administering oseltamivir (Tamiflu, Roche Pharmaceuticals, Nutley, NJ) or other antivirals is not recommended for several reasons (**Box 2**).

Box 2
Reasons not to use oseltamivir for the treatment of Canine Influenza H3N8

1. Timing of use. Oseltamivir acts by trapping viruses in infected cells. It must be administered very early, before the virus is widely spread in the body, to be of benefit. Most animals are presented to a veterinarian after this point.

2. Safety and efficacy. There have been no studies on the clinical use of oseltamivir in dogs.

3. Lack of need. Most dogs will recover from canine influenza with good supportive care.

4. Possible resistance. There is no system for detecting oseltamivir resistance in canine influenza should it appear.

5. Public health. Tamiflu overuse is being discouraged in both human and veterinary medicine. Should an influenza pandemic occur, antivirals will more likely be effective if they have not been overused.

Data from UC Davis Koret Shelter Medicine Program. Information—Canine influenza. May 2006. Available at: http://www.sheltermedicine.com/portal/is_canine_influenza_update.shtml#top3. Accessed July 30, 2008.

Prevention

As of yet there is no vaccine available to prevent canine influenza. The equine influenza vaccine should not be used on dogs.[44] It is not clear whether "antigenic drift" will be seen in the canine influenza virus as is seen in human seasonal influenza. This would necessitate regular updating of any vaccine to maintain its efficacy. Vaccinations for other canine respiratory diseases should be administered to maintain the health of the respiratory tract, and to help clarify when a canine influenza outbreak might be occurring.

Case Study: Canine Influenza Outbreak in Los Angeles County, 2007

A 5-month-old puppy of unknown origin presented at a veterinary clinic on July 10, 2007 with a fever of 104.5°F, nasal discharge, pneumonia, and vomiting. The puppy was placed in isolation and treated with intravenous fluids, antibiotics, a humidifier, and coupage. On July 13, the puppy was moved to an oxygen cage in the main treatment area, which was adjacent to the boarding section of the clinic. The puppy died soon after.

On July 17, clients began notifying the clinic of coughing in their dogs. The outbreak was reported by the owner of the practice to Los Angeles County Veterinary Public Health, which assisted with diagnostics. Approximately 43 dogs were identified in the outbreak, over a period of 17 days (**Fig. 2**). Most cases (72%) had been boarded at the clinic before onset, while others were outpatients or had contact with a boarded dog. Seven cases had thoracic radiographs performed, of which four had bronchopneumonia. The vast majority of cases were prescribed an oral antibiotic. Only the index case was hospitalized. Serology was performed on six coughing dogs and four healthy dogs that had been in the boarding area. Interestingly, all four healthy dogs were seronegative, despite likely exposure. Five of the six coughing dogs tested were seropositive. Two of these five had a convalescent serum sample drawn 3 weeks later, which revealed a fourfold rise in titer in both cases. Nasal and pharyngeal swabs of two other coughing dogs were negative by PCR.

The clinic closed their boarding section to new admissions for 20 days beginning on August 1st. Surgeries and outpatient appointments were not cancelled. Staff were assigned to work in either the back of the clinic (where hospitalized patients were

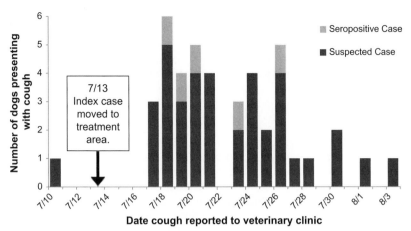

Fig. 2. Epidemic curve of canine influenza H3N8 at a veterinary clinic in Los Angeles County, 2007.

located), or the front, (where outpatients were seen), and were not allowed to cross between the two sections. The lobby was mopped with disinfectant six times daily. All fomites commonly touched by people (like phones, doorknobs, faucet handles, countertop pens, and door face plates) were disinfected four times daily during the outbreak and for 1 month after. The comprehensive approach this clinic took to infection control helped limit the outbreak to less than a month, despite the ongoing caseload in the practice. They reported almost no loss of clientele.

Canine Influenza H3N8 and Public Health

Canine influenza H3N8 is not considered to be zoonotic. However, because it has already exhibited a change in species specificity by jumping from horses to dogs, any human illness following contact with ill dogs should be noted and public health authorities alerted.

INFLUENZA IN CATS AND DOGS—GENERAL RECOMMENDATIONS

1. Know about the options for influenza testing. Serologic and PCR testing for canine influenza A H3N8 testing is commercially available. Tests for other influenza strains may possibly be performed by diagnostics labs through special arrangement.
2. Follow the news and the latest research. Two examples of free, online sources are:
   a. Emerging Infectious Disease, a free journal published by the Centers for Disease Control and Prevention (CDC) can be found at: http://www.cdc.gov/ncidod/eid.
   b. ProMed mail. Human, animal, and plant outbreak news from all over the world e-mailed daily, from the International Society for Infectious Diseases. http://www.promedmail.org/.
3. Know your local and state public health authorities.
4. Practice basic zoonosis control within your clinic. The National Association of State Public Health Veterinarians (NASPHV) has written a compendium of standards: http://www.nasphv.org/Documents/VeterinaryPrecautions.pdf.

5. Have a plan for handing outbreaks within your clinic. The Model Infection Control Plan for Veterinary Practices from the NASPHV can be found at: http://www.nasphv.org/documentsCompendia.html.
6. Educate staff and clients about influenza to minimize unreasonable fears. The most useful step you can take is to be knowledgeable and to have clear-cut recommendations ready.

SUMMARY

Since 2004, highly pathogenic avian influenza H5N1 has infected cats and dogs, primarily though ingestion of raw infected birds. The virus also spread from cat-to-cat in isolated cases. The virus apparently cannot be transmitted dog-to-dog. No cases of zoonotic transmission from a cat or dog have been reported. There is one report of illness in dogs due to avian H3N2 virus; these cases, reported from South Korea, were most likely acquired through consumption of raw infected poultry. Canine influenza H3N8 is the only influenza fully adapted to, and highly contagious among, dogs. It is the strain most veterinarians are likely to encounter in practice.

ACKNOWLEDGMENTS

Many thanks to Mary Trainor, Dr. Karen Ehnert, DVM, MPVM, Dr. Patrick Ryan, DVM, MPH, Kathryn Farrar, Anthony Moreno, and Dr. Rosalie Trevejo, DVM, MPH, for their patient help in reviewing this manuscript.

REFERENCES

1. Horimoto T, Kawaoka Y. Pandemic threat posed by avian influenza A viruses. Clin Microbiol Rev 2001;14(1):129–49.
2. Spickler AR. Influenza. The center for food security and the public's health. Available at: http://www.cfsph.iastate.edu/Factsheets/pdfs/influenza.pdf. August 6, 2007. Accessed May 25, 2008.
3. Bieker JM, Souza CA, Oberst RD. Inactivation of various influenza strains to model avian influenza (bird flu) with various disinfectant chemistries. Available at: http://www.prod.sandia.gov/cgi-bin/techlib/access-control.pl/2005/057633.pdf. Accessed May 23, 2008.
4. Ghedin E, Sengamalay NA, Shumway M, et al. Large-scale sequencing of human influenza reveals the dynamic nature of viral genome evolution. Nature 2005; 437(7062):1162–6.
5. Liu JP. Avian influenza—a pandemic waiting to happen. J Microbiol Immunol Infect 2006;39:4–10.
6. Callan RJ, Early G, Kida H, et al. The appearance of H3 viruses in seals. J Gen Virol 1995;76:199–203.
7. The Merck veterinary manual. Available at: http://www.merckvetmanual.com/mvm/index.jsp. Accessed May 29, 2008.
8. Morens DM, Fauci AS. The 1918 influenza pandemic: insights for the 21st century. J Infect Dis 2007;195:1018–28.
9. Taubenberger JK, Morens DM. 1918 Influenza: the mother of all pandemics. Emerg Infect Dis 2006;12(1):15–22.
10. Peiris JSM, Jong de, Guan Y. Avian influenza virus (H5N1): a threat to human health. Clin Microbiol Rev 2007;20(2):243–67.
11. Songserm T, Amonsin A, Jam-on R, et al. Fatal avian influenza A H5N1 in a dog. Emerg Infect Dis 2006;12(11):1744–7.

12. U.S. Department of Agriculture. Animal plant health inspection service veterinary services. Recent Spread Of Highly Pathogenic (H5N1) Avian Influenza in Birds. May 22, 2006. Available at: http://www.aphis.usda.gov/vs/ceah/cei/taf/emerginganimalhealthissues_files/hpai_recentspread.pdf. Accessed May 29, 2008.
13. Chotpitayasunondh T, Ungshusak K, Hanshaoworakul W, et al. Human disease from influenza A (H5N1), Thailand, 2004. Emerg Infect Dis 2005;11(2):201–9.
14. Van Riel D, Munster VJ, de Wit E, et al. Human and avian influenza viruses target different cells in the lower respiratory tract of humans and other mammals. Am J Pathol 2007;171(1):1215–23.
15. Paniker CKJ, Nair CMG. Infection with A2 Hong Kong influenza virus in domestic cats. Bull World Health Organ 1970;43:859–62.
16. Paniker CKJ, Nair CMG. Experimental infection of animals with influenza-virus types A and B. Bull World Health Organ 1972;47:461–3.
17. Hinshaw VS, Webster RG, Easterday BC, et al. Replication of avian influenza A viruses in mammals. Infect Immun 1981;34(2):354–61.
18. World Health Organization. Avian influenza A (H5N1)—update 28: reports of infection in domestic cats (Thailand), situation (human) in Thailand, situation (poultry) in Japan and China. Available at: http://www.who.int/csr/don/2004_02_20/en/. Feb 20, 2004. Accessed April 20, 2008.
19. Li Y. The first finding of tiger influenza by virus isolation and specific gene amplification (China). ProMed Mail 2004. Available at: www.promedmail.org. Archive number 20041023.2873. Accessed April 20, 2008.
20. Keawcharoen J, Oraveerakul K, Kuiken T, et al. Avian influenza H5N1 in tigers and leopards. Emerg Infect Dis 2004;10(12):2189–91.
21. Thanawongnuwech R, Amonsin A, Tantilertcharoen R, et al. Probable tiger-to-tiger transmission of avian influenza H5N1. Emerg Infect Dis 2005;11(5):699–701.
22. Songserm T, Amonsin A, Rungroj J, et al. Avian influenza H5N1 in a naturally infected domestic cat. Emerg Infect Dis 2006;12(4):681–3.
23. Yingst SL, Saad MD, Felt SA. Qinghai-like H5N1 from domestic cats, northern Iraq. Emerg Infect Dis 2006;12(8):1295–7.
24. Weber S, Harder T, Starick E, et al. Molecular analysis of highly pathogenic avian influenza of subtype H5N1 isolated from wild birds and mammals in northern Germany. J Gen Virol 2007;88:554–8.
25. Leschnik M, Weikel J, Möstl K, et al. Subclinical infection with avian influenza A (H5N1) virus in cats. Emerg Infect Dis 2007;13(2):243–7.
26. MacKenzie D. Deadly H5N1 may be brewing in cats. New Sci 2007;193(2588):6–7.
27. Kuiken T, Rimmelzwaan G, Van Riel D, et al. Avian H5N1 influenza in cats. Science 2004;306:241.
28. Rimmelzwaan GF, Van Riel D, Baars M, et al. Influenza A virus (H5N1) infection in cats causes systemic diseases with potential novel routes of virus spread within and between hosts. Am J Pathol 2006;168(1):176–83.
29. Giese M, Harder TC, Teifke JP, et al. Experimental infection and natural contact exposure of dogs with avian influenza virus (H5N1). Emerg Infect Dis 2008;14(2):308–10.
30. Vahlenkamp TW, Harder TC, et al. Protection of cats against lethal influenza H5N1 challenge infection. J Gen Virol 2008;89:968–74.
31. Dougherty C. Bird flu fears and new rules rattle German pet lovers. New York Times online. March 5, 2006. Available at: http://www.nytimes.com/2006/03/05/international/europe/05flu.html.

32. Altman LK. Article on bird flu criticizes effort to monitor cats and dogs. The New York Times online. April 6, 2006. Available at: http://www.nytimes.com/2006/04/06/world/europe/06cat.html?_r=1&;oref=slogin. Accessed April 6, 2006.

33. Madhavan HN, Agarwai SC. Sero-epidemiology of human and canine influenza in Pondicherry, south India, during 1971–1974. Indian J Med Res 1976;64(6):835–40.

34. Mail ProMed. Officials say Azeri dog dies of bird flu. Available at: http://www.promedmail.org. March 16, 2006. archive number 20060316.0818. Accessed May 25, 2008.

35. Butler D. Thai dogs carry bird-flu virus, but will they spread it? Nature 2006;439:773.

36. The Nation, Bangkok's independent newspaper. Deadly virus: dog contracts avian flu. Available at: http://nationmultimedia.com/option/print.php?newsid=30012411. August 31, 2006. Accessed September 6, 2006.

37. Maas R, Tacken M, Ruuls L, et al. Avian influenza (H5N1) susceptibility and receptors in dogs. Emerg Infect Dis 2007;13(8):1219–21.

38. Song D, Kang B, Lee C, et al. Transmission of avian influenza virus (H3N2) to dogs. Emerg Infect Dis 2008;14(5):741–6.

39. Crawford PC, Dubovi EJ, Castleman WL, et al. Transmission of equine influenza virus to dogs. Science 2005;310:482–5.

40. American Veterinary Medical Association. Control of canine influenza in dogs—questions, answers, and interim guidelines. Available at: http://www.avma.org/public_health/influenza/canine_guidelines.asp. December 1, 2005. Accessed May 1, 2008.

41. International Conference on Emerging Infectious Diseases—Press Release. Canine influenza was around as early as 1999. Available at: http://www.asm.org/ASM/files/LeftMarginHeaderList/DOWNLOADFILENAME/000000002750/dog%20flu.pdf. March 18, 2008. Accessed April 16, 2008.

42. Daly JM, Blunden AS, MacRae S, et al. Transmission of equine influenza to English foxhounds. Emerg Infect Dis 2008;14(3):461–4.

43. Long MT, Gibbs EPJ, Crawford PC, et al. Comparison of virus replication and clinical disease in horses inoculated with equine or canine influenza viruses. Presented at: Immunobiology of Influenza Virus Infection: Approaches for an Emerging Zoonotic Disease. Athens (GA), July 29–31, 2007.

44. UC Davis Koret Shelter Medicine Program. Information – Canine influenza. Available at: http://www.sheltermedicine.com/portal/is_canine_influenza_update.shtml#top3. May 2006. Accessed July 30, 08.

45. U.S. Environmental Protection Agency. Disposal of domestic birds infected by avian influenza – an overview of considerations and options. Available at: http://www.epa.gov/epaoswer/homeland/flu.pdf. August 11, 2006. Accessed May 25, 2008.

46. Bridges CB, Kuehnert MJ, Hall CB. Transmission of influenza: implications for control in health care settings. Clinical Infectious Diseases 2003;371094–101.

47. U.S. Pandemic Influenza Website. Control of pandemic flu virus on environmental surfaces in homes and public places. Available at: http://www.pandemicflu.gov/plan/individual/panfacts.html. Accessed May 25, 2008.

48. Canadian Food Inspection Agency. Pathogen data safety sheet – highly pathogenic avian influenza (HPAI). Available at: http://www.inspection.gc.ca/english/sci/bio/anima/disemala/avflue.shtml. 2005. Accessed May 23, 2008.

49. U.S. Pandemic Influenza Website. Is there a risk for becoming infected with avian influenza by eating poultry? Available at: http://www.pandemicflu.gov/faq/foodsafety/1095.html. Accessed May 25, 2008.

Emerging Tick-borne Diseases

Curtis L. Fritz, DVM, MPVM, PhD

KEYWORDS

- Tick-borne diseases • Lyme disease
- Rocky mountain spotted fever • Zoonoses • Ehrlichiosis

In 1992, the Institute of Medicine (IOM) published the first treatise on "emerging infections," a sobering warning of the resilience and plasticity of microbial organisms to adapt rapidly to changing environments and evolutionary pressures and to exploit newly created niches.[1] This prescient publication anticipated numerous types of public health threats, including diseases that were truly new (eg, sudden acute respiratory syndrome), were newly described (eg, hantavirus cardiopulmonary syndrome), had expanded their geographic endemicity (eg, West Nile virus), or had increased their pathogenicity (eg, methicillin-resistant *Staphylococcus aureus*). Several diseases also have "emerged" through facilitated transmission as a consequence of increased numbers and density of susceptible individuals (eg, opportunistic infections of HIV patients), permeation of geographic barriers (eg, H5:N1 avian influenza), or malicious intentional dissemination (eg, *Bacillus anthracis*).

Vector-borne diseases are particularly prone to the environmental pressures that contribute to changes in the ecology and the emergence of disease pathogens. These diseases are defined by and are dependent on climate and habitat that are compatible with the biologic needs of the microbiologic pathogens, their arthropod vector(s), and their mammalian reservoir(s). Ecologic changes on the macro scale (eg, global climate change) or micro scale (eg, suburban development) can alter established geographic and epidemiologic domains of vector-borne diseases.

Emerging infections are not a concern that is isolated to public health. The IOM report emphasized that "[t]he significance of zoonoses in the emergence of human infections cannot be overstated." Indeed, the complex cycles of vector-borne zoonoses often include multiple mammalian and non-mammalian vertebrate and invertebrate species. Humans and domestic canids are particularly intertwined in their respective roles in and risks for diseases transmitted by ticks. In addition to being susceptible to tick-borne diseases, dogs may serve as reservoirs for human pathogens, as definitive feeding hosts for vector ticks, as mechanical transporters of ticks, and as sentinel indicators of regional disease risk. Conversely, in the absence of centralized reporting for most canine diseases, surveillance and other data collected for

Division of Communicable Disease Control, California Department of Public Health, 1616 Capitol Avenue, MS 7307, P.O. Box 997377, Sacramento, CA 95899-7377, USA
E-mail address: cfritz@cdph.ca.gov

Vet Clin Small Anim 39 (2009) 265–278
doi:10.1016/j.cvsm.2008.10.019
0195-5616/08/$ – see front matter © 2009 Elsevier Inc. All rights reserved.

vetsmall.theclinics.com

tick-borne diseases in humans can lend insight into risks for veterinary patients. Surveillance, diagnosis, treatment, and prevention of tick-borne diseases in humans and dogs can yield mutually beneficial information for public and veterinary health.

This article highlights the epidemiology of tick-borne zoonoses of concern to humans and domestic pets in North America. Because a comprehensive review of these diseases is not possible in this brief space, readers desiring detailed information on clinical signs, diagnosis, and management are directed to recently published reviews and standard texts.[2–6]

TICKS

Ticks are arthropods belonging to the order Arachnida. They are free living but require a blood meal during at least one life stage. "Soft" ticks (family: Argasidae) attach to the host, complete feeding within a few minutes, and promptly detach. "Hard" ticks (family: Ixodidae) are protracted feeders and remain attached for up to several days before reaching repletion. Successive blood meals on different hosts permit the transmission of blood-borne pathogens from one host to another. Ticks species with catholic feeding preferences can transmit microbes from evolutionarily commensal reservoir species (eg, rodents) to incidental susceptible species (eg, humans). The risk of disease transmission therefore is determined by the prevalence of infectious ticks—a function of the number and infection prevalence of the pathogen's reservoir host—and by the likelihood of an encounter between an infected tick and a susceptible host—a function of both the numbers of ticks and susceptible hosts within a fixed area and their respective behaviors.

Approximately 400 species of ixodid ticks occur worldwide, but fewer than 100 occur in North America. Only a dozen or so North American tick species parasitize humans or dogs with any frequency and are known to transmit micro-organisms of medical significance. Usually only one or two species of tick can acquire, maintain, and transmit a given pathogen. Therefore, the distribution of disease risk is restricted by the necessity for sympatric coexistence of the microbial pathogen, a competent vector tick, a reservoir host, and a susceptible host. The risk of disease parallels the geographic and seasonal distribution of ticks; therefore, veterinarians should educate themselves about which tick species are present within their practice area. Veterinarians can consult entomologists at their state universities, county or state departments of public health, or local mosquito and vector control districts for information on tick prevalence and for assistance in identifying ticks recovered from their patients.

The regions of tick-borne disease risk are not necessarily static. The spatial and temporal boundaries of risk for a given tick-borne disease may fluctuate over the short or long term as favorable conditions expand or contract. Transient meteorologic phenomena in endemic areas (eg, a wet, mild winter) can extend the number of months in which ticks are active in a given year. Protracted or permanent climatologic change can transform previously nonendemic areas to habitat favorable to ticks (eg, warmer temperatures in higher elevations or upper latitudes). Similarly, the spatial dimension of a risk area may change physically through human encroachment into or modification of existing tick habitat or change practically by susceptible individuals increasing behaviors that facilitate contact with questing ticks. Many "emerging" tick-borne diseases may represent micro-organism–tick–mammal disease cycles that are not truly new but have been newly discovered and described as a consequence of direct or indirect changes in the risk area and, consequently, the empiric morbidity.

LYME BORRELIOSIS

Disease caused by spirochetes of the genus *Borrelia* has been recognized in Europe since the early 1900s. Disease caused by a *Borrelia* indigenous to North America was first reported in 1977 among a localized cluster of patients diagnosed with juvenile rheumatoid arthritis.[7] The spirochete, *Borrelia burgdorferi*, described in 1982, encompasses four groups, of which Group 1, *B. burgdorferi* sensu stricto, is the principal pathogenic strain in North America.[8,9] A myriad of clinical manifestations now is recognized, including dermatologic (characteristic erythema migrans rash), neurologic (encephalitis, meningitis, radiculoneuropathy), cardiologic (atrioventricular conduction deficits), and rheumatologic (mono- or oligoarticular arthritis).

B. burgdorferi is transmitted to mammalian hosts by ixodid ticks. *Ixodes scapularis* is the principal vector in the northeastern and upper Midwestern United States; *I. pacificus* is the vector along the Pacific Coast. Distribution of favorable tick habitat (temperate, humid forests near large bodies of water), feeding hosts (deer), and reservoir hosts (rodents) determine distribution of disease. In 2006, approximately 95% of the nearly 20,000 cases of Lyme borreliosis reported in the United States were in residents of the upper midwestern (Minnesota and Wisconsin), northeastern (New York, New Hampshire, Pennsylvania, Vermont, Rhode Island, Connecticut, Massachusetts, and Maine), and mid-Atlantic (Maryland, New Jersey, and Delaware) states.[10] Expanding human populations and the resultant environmental alterations in the twentieth century probably contributed to defining these areas of endemicity. Areas that until the early 1900s were heavily wooded were converted to agrarian land that reduced habitat for deer. As populations of deer (and their ticks) plummeted, *Ixodes muris*, a one-host tick that feeds on rodents, came to dominate the acarologic landscape. In the mid-twentieth century, agriculture succumbed to suburbanization and reforestation, leading to a resurgence of deer and their attendant ectoparasites, chiefly *I. scapularis*, in areas that overlapped with human habitation. The epidemic of Lyme borreliosis apparent in the late twentieth century reflected this potentiation of transmission in the peri-residential environment and also increased recognition among health care providers and the expanded availability of often highly sensitive but poorly specific diagnostic assays.

Dogs are susceptible to infection with *B. burgdorferi*, but clinical disease generally is milder, narrower in scope, and less frequent than in humans.[11] Only about 5% to 10% of dogs exposed to infected ticks develop clinical borreliosis.[12] Clinical borreliosis manifests chiefly as polyarthritis approximately 2 to 6 months after exposure and typically is self-limited. A small percentage of dogs also develop a protein-losing glomerulopathy.[13] Serologic studies have documented immunologic evidence of borreliosis in cats, but clinical illness is rare.[14]

Aside from their shared susceptibility, dogs contribute little to the public health concerns of Lyme borreliosis. Dogs are not an efficient reservoir for the spirochete, nor are they an important or preferred feeding host for *Ixodes* ticks. It has been hypothesized that dogs may introduce ticks into the peri-domestic environment from an outdoor, distant source. Although in theory a partially fed tick may present a slightly increased risk of disease transmission (because spirochetes already have migrated from the midgut to the salivary glands), ticks generally do not re-feed if detached before repletion. Because of their frequent encounters with ticks and ready seroconversion, dogs have been proposed as sentinels for humans' risk of Lyme borreliosis.[15] Targeted research studies using domestic dogs can help sketch broad areas where *B. burgdorferi* is present, but, because of the highly focal distribution of vector ticks, a reliable range of endemicity is delineated better by surveillance of ticks and natural rodent hosts than by serologic or clinical evidence from incidentally infected hosts.

The diagnosis of Lyme borreliosis in both humans and dogs can be challenging. Clinical signs often are nonspecific and variable. Culture of the spirochete requires special media over a lengthy incubation period and often is unrewarding. Assays for circulating antibodies remain the most common means of laboratory confirmation despite recognized shortcomings.[16] Enzyme immunoassays (EIA) and immunofluorescent assays (IFA) based on the whole cell or subunits of the spirochete generally lack specificity. The US Centers for Disease Control and Prevention recommends a two-step procedure in which specimens yielding a positive or equivocal result on a screening EIA or IFA are confirmed by Western immunoblotting using specific interpretation criteria.[17] Recently developed assays that use IR6, an antigen that is highly conserved among *Borrelia* spp and is expressed transiently only in actively infected mammalian hosts, may make more specific screening tests possible.[18,19] A commercial test that uses a recombinant form of the IR6 (C6) seems to be more specific than whole-cell sonicates.[20] Nevertheless, seropositivity may not indicate active infection and should not be used as the sole criterion for diagnosis. Interpretation of laboratory results and decisions regarding treatment should be based on the likelihood of Lyme borreliosis in the patient, including clinical, laboratory, and epidemiologic factors (eg, region of country, outdoor activities, history of tick bite). Routine treatment of seropositive asymptomatic dogs generally is unwarranted, because most dogs do not develop clinical signs, illness often is self-limited, and injudicious antimicrobial treatment may contribute to emergence of antibiotic resistance in other flora with zoonotic potential.[21,22]

RICKETTSIOSES

Obligately intracellular bacteria in the order *Rickettsiales* cause several tick-borne diseases of human and veterinary medical importance. The family Rickettsiaceae contains bacteria of the genus *Rickettsia*, including *R. rickettsii*, the agent of Rocky Mountain spotted fever (RMSF). The family Anaplasmataceae encompasses several pathogens of humans and animals in the genera *Ehrlichia* and *Anaplasma* that formerly were grouped under the broad term "ehrlichiosis."

Rocky Mountain Spotted Fever

R. rickettsii is one of more than a dozen species of *Rickettsia* in the spotted fever group (SFG); these rickettsiae are closely related to typhus group *Rickettsia* spp (eg, *R. typhi*) but are distinct from other rickettsiae. RMSF is the most frequently reported rickettsial illness in humans in the United States; about 2300 cases were reported in 2006.[10] RMSF in humans is characterized by high fever, myalgia, severe headache, and a petechial or maculopapular rash of the extremities, including palms and soles. Case-fatality of untreated patients is 3% to 5%. The initial clinical signs of RMSF in dogs resemble those in humans: fever, myalgias, and petechiae/ecchymoses, chiefly of the mucous membranes. Damage to the vascular endothelium leads to hypoalbuminemia and development of extremital and cerebral edema. Hypotension, shock, and renal hypoperfusion and failure also may occur.

RMSF cases are distributed throughout much of the United States because of the ranges of its two principal tick vectors: *Dermacentor variabilis* (the American dog tick) in the southeastern and south central states, where more than 80% of cases occur, and *D. andersonii* (Rocky Mountain wood tick) in the Rocky Mountains and the Northwest. Other tick species such as *Amblyomma americanum* (the lone star tick) and *Rhipicephalus sanguineus* (the brown dog tick) also can occasionally transmit *R. rickettsii*. *Rh. sanguineus*, a one-host tick whose preferred host is canids, was implicated recently in an outbreak of RMSF among humans and domestic dogs in Arizona,[23–25] a state where RMSF is rarely reported and *Dermacentor* ticks are uncommon. Investigators hypothesized that domestic dogs contributed directly to the outbreak by transporting ticks to the peri-domestic environment, supporting large populations of ticks in close proximity to human habitation, and possibly serving as a reservoir for the *Rickettsia*. Evaluation of archived sera indicate that free-roaming canids in Arizona were exposed to *R. rickettsii* at least a decade before this outbreak.[26]

Serologic assays are the most widely available laboratory diagnostic. Because of considerable cross-reactivity between SFG rickettsiae and the variable specificity of commercial assays,[27] documentation of a fourfold change in serum antibody titer between acute and convalescent specimens—ideally, submitted simultaneously and tested in parallel—is recommended. To avoid delay in initiating treatment, a provisional diagnosis may be made based on clinical compatibility, history and species of tick infestation, and epidemiologic indicators such as region of the country and season of year (chiefly late spring to early autumn). A single elevated IgM titer in a clinically compatible patient may be sufficient for confirmation. In contrast, because canine IgG to *Rickettsia* spp may persist for up to 10 months,[27–29] detection of IgG alone may not be clinically relevant.

Ehrlichioses and Anaplasmosis

Zoonotic members of the family Anaplasmataceae are pathogens of leukocytes and usually are grouped based on their leukocytotropic propensity. Monocytotropic *Ehrlichia* spp include closely related agents of human (*E. chaffeensis*) and canine (*E. canis*) ehrlichiosis. Members of the former granulocytotropic *E. phagocytophila* group—including pathogens of humans (human granulocytic ehrlichiosis agent), ruminants (*E. phagocytophila*), equids (*E. equi*), and other mammals—recently were reclassified collectively as *Anaplasma phagocytophilum*.[30] (A closely related thrombocytotropic pathogen of dogs [*A. platys*] has not demonstrated zoonotic potential.)

E. canis was the first of the monocytic ehrlichioses to be identified, described in dogs in Algeria in 1937. Canine monocytic ehrlichiosis came to the attention of Western nations in the 1960s when several hundred military dogs died of the disease while serving in Vietnam.[31] Monocytic ehrlichiosis in humans was first recognized in the United States in the 1980s and initially was attributed to *E. canis*.[32] Subsequent investigation identified a closely related but distinct rickettsia, given the name *E. chaffeensis*.[33] Despite profound serologic cross-reactivity among patients and greater than 98% homology based on 16S rRNA, *E. canis* and *E. chaffeensis* seem to be epidemiologically distinct. *E. chaffeensis* is restricted chiefly to the southeastern and south-central United States, deer are the likely reservoir host, and *A. americanum* is the principal tick vector; whereas *E. canis* is distributed worldwide, dogs serve as the reservoir, and *Rh. sanguineus* is the vector. Although dogs may be infected incidentally with *E. chaffeensis*, they seem to have limited susceptibility and no role in its maintenance.[34] Similarly, *E. canis* infection of humans is restricted to a few reported cases in South America.[35]

Another member of the *Ehrlichia* group, *E. ewingii*, has been identified as a pathogen of both dogs and humans. *E. ewingii* shares 98% genetic homology with *E. canis* and *E. chaffeensis*[36] and seems to resemble *E. chaffeensis* in its geographic distribution (the southeastern and south-central United States), tick vector (*A. americanum*), and seasonality (spring to autumn). *E. ewingii* differs from other members of this group in that it is chiefly granulocytotropic.[37] Canine granulocytic ehrlichiosis was first described in a dog from Arkansas in 1971,[38] and *E. ewingii* was identified as the etiologic agent in 1992.[36] The first report of *E. ewingii* infections in humans was published in 1999,[37] describing four male patients from Missouri who presented with histories of tick bites and clinical illness consistent with ehrlichiosis; three of these patients were being treated with immunosuppressive therapy. The full contribution of *E. ewingii* to human morbidity remains undetermined but seems to be low.

A. phagocytophilum is a granulocytotropic rickettsia distinct from the *E. canis/chaffeensis* group. Evidence of natural infection with *A. phagocytophilum* has been identified in humans, horses, dogs, small ruminants, and some wild mammals.[39–42] Rare cases of a mild and self-limited infection with *A. phagocytophilum* have been reported in cats from the northeastern United States.[43] Because the rodent reservoirs (*Peromyscus* mice, *Neotoma* rats) and tick vectors (*Ixodes* spp) for *A. phagocytophilum* in the United States are similar to those for Lyme borreliosis, it shares similar geographic distribution and seasonality—that is, the northeastern and upper midwestern states from spring to early summer and autumn. *Ixodes* ticks can be coinfected with both organisms,[44,45] and concurrent infections with *A. phagocytophilum* and *B. burgdorferi* have been observed in humans.[46,47] The clinical likelihood and significance of coinfection with these pathogens in other species is unknown.

The distinctive leukocytotropisms of *Ehrlichia* spp and *A. phagocytophilum* offer a means of provisionally diagnosing and differentiating infections with these rickettsiae. During the acute phase of illness, binary fission of the rickettsiae within the phagosome produces membrane-bound intracytoplasmic aggregates called "morulae." Morulae in circulating leukocytes can be observed directly in Romanovsky-stained blood or buffy coat smears. Identifying the leukocytic cell line containing morulae can narrow the list of possible rickettsial pathogens, but different rickettsia species within a leukocytotropic group (eg, granulocytotropic *E. ewingii* and *A. phagocytophilum*) cannot be discriminated further based on morulae prevalence or morphology. Although observation of intraleukocytic morulae is highly specific when performed by a trained microbiologist, it offers only low-to-moderate sensitivity, depending on when the specimen was collected and the type and proportion of leukocytes infected. Typically, both the proportion of patients in whom morulae are observed (< 5%–10% for monocytic morulae[48,49] and 25% for granulocytic morulae)[50] and the proportion of leukocytes containing morulae during active infection (1%–2% for monocytes[32] and up to 80% for neutrophils)[39,51] are quite low. Therefore, serology remains the principal, but not definitive, method for diagnosis. Cross-reactivity between ehrlichiae and *A. phagocytophilum* is common in both canine and human sera.[52,53] Differentiation may be confirmed by more specific assays (Western immunoblotting or polymerase chain reaction), when available, or may be inferred through demonstration of a fourfold change in titer between acute and convalescent specimens.

TULAREMIA

"Tularemia" is a general term for the myriad of clinical manifestations that can occur following infection with the gram-negative bacillus, *Francisella tularensis*. *F. tularensis* is distributed widely throughout North America, because of multiple mammalian reservoir species, the persistence of the bacteria in the environment, and several competent arthropod vectors. Four species of ticks—*D. andersonii*, *D. variabilis*, *D. occidentalis*, and *A. americanum*—are recognized as true biologic vectors and reservoirs for *F. tularensis* at least one of which exists in almost any given region of the United States. Other routes of transmission include handling or ingestion of tissues from an infected mammal (principally lagomorphs), ingestion of or inoculation with contaminated water through a break in the skin or mucous membrane, inhalation of contaminated dust, and mechanical transmission by other biting arthropods such as deer flies (*Crysops* spp) and mosquitoes. Because of the potential for respiratory exposure and the low inoculum (10–50 organisms) necessary to effect infection, *F. tularensis* is considered a Category A potential bioterrorism agent.[54]

The route of infection generally determines the scope of clinical manifestations. Humans most commonly are infected through direct contact or tick bite, leading to an ulceropapular lesion at the site of inoculation and localized lymphadenomegaly. The ulceroglandular form predominates in humans, but typhoidal, glandular, oculoglandular, and pneumonic forms also occur. The spectrum of illness in domestic animals seems to be much narrower. Dogs are exposed most frequently via tick bite but seem to be relatively resistant to infection; transient mild fever and anorexia have been reported.[55] Infection in cats is more severe; because cats are likely to be infected through predation and consumption of infected rodents or rabbits,[56] lymphadenopathy and ulcerations of the oropharynx are the most frequently observed signs.[57]

Infected dogs and cats may present a low risk of transmission to humans. Bites or scratches from cats have been associated with more than 50 human cases of tularemia.[58,59] Dogs are unlikely to serve as a direct source of transmission but may facilitate exposure by bringing infectious ticks, tissues (eg, rabbit carcasses), or water (eg, a saturated coat from a contaminated lake) into the peri-domestic environment. The bacterial load in suppurative lesions is low, but because only a few organisms are necessary to cause infection, veterinary staff should use barrier protection when handling patients suspected of having tularemia. Cultures and necropsies of suspect patients should be performed only in Biosafety Level 3 facilities.

POSSIBLE EMERGING TICK-BORNE ZOONOSES

Several pathogens recently have been identified for which transmission by ticks or the zoonotic potential have yet to be established. Some members of the genus *Bartonella* have long been associated with transmission by biting arthropods; for example, *B. quintana*, the agent of trench fever in humans, is transmitted by the human body louse. *B. henselae* is a widespread commensal bacterium among healthy domestic cats but causes bacillary angiomatosis ("cat scratch disease") in humans who are bitten or scratched. Fleas harbor the organism, and contamination of skin breaks with flea excrement, rather than the feline scratch per se, seems to be required for infection. *B. henselae* also has been identified in attached and questing ticks,[60–62] but their competence as vectors has yet to be verified.[63] Infection with *B. vinsonii* has been associated with valvular endocarditis in some dogs and humans.[64–66] Serum antibodies to *B. vinsonii* have been detected in numerous surveys of both healthy and diseased wild and domestic canids.[67–71] Often these canids had concomitant heavy tick infestations and seroreactivity to other tick-borne pathogens (eg, *E. canis*), but at present there is no direct evidence that ticks are a competent vector of *B. vinsonii*.

A skin rash resembling the erythema migrans lesion of Lyme borreliosis has been described in residents of southern and central parts of the United States where *Ixodes* ticks and *B. burgdorferi* are rare.[72,73] The disease Southern tick-associated rash illness (STARI) is associated with bites from the lone star tick, *Amblyomma americanum*,[74] and has been linked provisionally to infection with *Borrelia lonestari*.[75] Human patients who have STARI show no serologic cross-reactivity on whole-cell and C6 ELISAs for *B. burgdorferi*.[76,77] Experimentally inoculated beagles developed detectable antibodies, but *B. lonestari* could not be re-isolated from blood.[78]

White-tailed deer are the only other vertebrate in which natural infection with *B. lonestari* has been identified.[79]

Three species of *Babesia* (*B. canis*, *B. gibsoni*, and *B. conradae*), an intraerythrocytic protozoan, have been described from North American dogs.[80,81] Although *B. gibsoni* is transmitted principally by ticks, contact transmission also has been strongly suggested, particularly among fighting breeds.[82,83] Despite a close phylogenetic relationship between *B. conradae* and *B. duncani*, a human piroplasm,[84] neither *B. conradae* nor other canine *Babesia* spp seem to be zoonotic.

PREVENTION

The simple and often singular mechanism by which tick-borne diseases are transmitted (viz, by tick bite) permits a multitude of avenues for prevention. No one technique is invariably effective, however, so an integrated program of several preventive components is desirable to maximize protection from infection.

Environmental modification through landscape management (eg, removal of leaf litter) or reduction in feeding hosts (eg, culling deer) can reduce tick populations but generally is impractical over the expansive area needed to be effective. Area application of acaricides can substantially reduce tick abundance around residential property but requires frequent re-application and may pose health risks for incidentally exposed nontarget animals. In contrast, topical acaricides directed at tick feeding hosts (eg, deer feeding stations, rodent bait boxes) reduce the concentration of chemical needed, but still require frequent visits to the stations by a large proportion of the targeted mammal population.

Susceptible individuals can alter their behavior and activities to limit the opportunity for contact with ticks. Simply stated, bites from ticks can be prevented by avoiding areas where ticks are present. If traffic in tick habitats is desirable or otherwise unavoidable, owners and pets should limit contact with uncultivated grasses, bushes, and shrubs that may harbor questing ticks. Dogs should be kept on leash and maintained in the middle of roads, paths, or other routes devoid of vegetation.

Ticks can be further dissociated from potential hosts through the use of physical or chemical barriers. Long pants and long-sleeved shirts can delay or confound the tick's attachment to the skin. Chemical repellents applied to clothing (eg, permethrin) or skin (eg, N,N-diethyl-meta-toluamide [DEET]) of humans can further deter questing ticks. The use of DEET on animals is not recommended and should be avoided. Control of ticks on dogs is facilitated by the availability of collars impregnated with permethrin or amitraz and topical solutions containing fipronil, imidacloprid, permethrin, or selamectin.[85–87] Amitraz-impregnated collars seem to be more effective in interrupting the tick life cycle and to be longer acting than topical applications of fipronil.[88] Amitraz and permethrin products are contraindicated for cats. Selamectin is effective in control of *Rh. sanguineus* and *D. variabilis* on dogs and is safe to use on cats.[89,90]

Dogs residing in areas highly endemic for Lyme borreliosis and subject to heavy tick infestation may benefit from immunization against *B. burgdorferi*. Reduced incidence of serum antibodies to *B. burgdorferi* and clinical borreliosis (ie, lameness) were observed among dogs vaccinated with a whole-cell bacterin.[91,92] Newer recombinant subunit vaccines based on the Osp A antigen of *B. burgdorferi* may interrupt transmission by complement-mediated lysis of the spirochete in the tick's gut soon after it begins its blood meal.[93] Vaccination against *B. burgdorferi* does not obviate the need for other measures to prevent tick bites, because the vaccine confers no cross-protection against other tick-borne pathogens.

Individuals should examine themselves, family members, and pets thoroughly after visiting tick-infested areas. Because *Ixodes* ticks do not transmit *B. burgdorferi* spirochetes efficiently until 24 to 48 hours after attachment, transmission of spirochetes pathogens can be prevented or interrupted by prompt recognition and removal of attached ticks.[94] A single dose of doxycycline administered within 72 hours of a recognized tick bite reduced infections with *B. burgdorferi* in humans,[95] but the efficacy and necessity of this prophylactic regimen for dogs and for other tick-borne pathogens has not been evaluated.

SUMMARY

Pets and their owners share susceptibility to several tick-borne diseases depending on their geographic location, season, and activities. When presented with a pet with possible tick-borne illness, veterinarians should take the opportunity to discuss the zoonotic disease risks with the owner. A comprehensive tick control program protects both pets and their owners by interrupting feeding opportunities for the tick and breaking the maintenance cycle of the pathogen. The veterinarian should consider the regional distribution of tick-borne diseases when formulating prevention strategies, diagnostic differentials, and therapeutic decisions. Because the complex cycles of microbial pathogens, vector ticks, environment, and mammalian hosts evolve continually and can lead to the emergence of tick-borne diseases in previously nonendemic areas, veterinarians should consult their local or state departments of public health for the most current information on which tick-borne diseases are of concern in their community.

REFERENCES

1. Lederberg J, Shope RE, Oaks SC Jr, editors. Emerging infections: microbial threats to health in the United States. Washington, DC: National Academy Press; 1992.
2. Green CE, editor. Infections diseases of the dog and cat. 3rd edition. St. Louis (MO): Elsevier, Inc; 2006.
3. Feldman KA. Tularemia. J Am Vet Med Assoc 2003;222(6):725–30.
4. Fritz CL, Kjemtrup AM. Lyme borreliosis. J Am Vet Med Assoc 2003;223(9): 1261–70.
5. Warner RD, Marsh WW. Rocky Mountain spotted fever. J Am Vet Med Assoc 2002; 221(10):1413–7.
6. McQuiston JH, McCall CL, Nicholson WL. Ehrlichiosis and related infections. J Am Vet Med Assoc 2003;223(12):1750–6.
7. Steere AC, Malawista SE, Snydman DR, et al. Lyme arthritis: an epidemic of oligoarticular arthritis in children and adults in three Connecticut communities. Arthritis Rheum 1977;20(1):7–17.
8. Mathiesen DA, Oliver JH Jr, Kolbert CP, et al. Genetic heterogeneity of *Borrelia burgdorferi* in the United States. J Infect Dis 1997;175(1):98–107.
9. Baranton G, Postic D, Saint Girons I, et al. Delineation of *Borrelia burgdorferi* sensu stricto, *Borrelia garinii* sp. nov., and group VS461 associated with Lyme borreliosis. Int J Syst Bacteriol 1992;42(3):378–83.
10. Centers for Disease Control and Prevention. Summary of notifiable diseases—United States, 2006. MMWR Morb Mortal Wkly Rep 2008;55(53):1–94.
11. Callister SM, Jobe DA, Schell RF, et al. Detection of borreliacidal antibodies in dogs after challenge with *Borrelia burgdorferi*-infected *Ixodes scapularis* ticks. J Clin Microbiol 2000;38(10):3670–4.

12. Levy SA, Magnarelli LA. Relationship between development of antibodies to *Borrelia burgdorferi* in dogs and the subsequent development of limb/joint borreliosis. J Am Vet Med Assoc 1992;200(3):344–7.

13. Grauer GF, Burgess EC, Cooley AJ, et al. Renal lesions associated with *Borrelia burgdorferi* infection in a dog. J Am Vet Med Assoc 1988;193(2):237–9.

14. Magnarelli LA, Anderson JF, Levine HR, et al. Tick parasitism and antibodies to *Borrelia burgdorferi* in cats. J Am Vet Med Assoc 1990;197(1):63–6.

15. Duncan AW, Correa MT, Levine JF, et al. The dog as a sentinel for human infection: prevalence of *Borrelia burgdorferi* C6 antibodies in dogs from southeastern and mid-Atlantic states. Vector Borne Zoonotic Dis 2005;5(2):101–9.

16. Tugwell P, Dennis DT, Weinstein A, et al. Laboratory evaluation in the diagnosis of Lyme disease. Ann Intern Med 1997;127(12):1109–23.

17. Centers for disease control and prevention. Recommendations for test performance and interpretation from the Second National Conference on Serologic Diagnosis of Lyme Disease. MMWR Morb Mortal Wkly Rep 1995;44(31):590–1.

18. Liang FT, Alvarez AL, Gu Y, et al. An immunodominant conserved region within the variable domain of VlsE, the variable surface antigen of *Borrelia burgdorferi*. J Immunol 1999;163(10):5566–73.

19. Liang FT, Jacobson RH, Straubinger RK, et al. Characterization of a *Borrelia burgdorferi* VlsE invariable region useful in canine Lyme disease serodiagnosis by enzyme-linked immunosorbent assay. J Clin Microbiol 2000;38(11):4160–6.

20. Liang FT, Steere AC, Marques AR, et al. Sensitive and specific serodiagnosis of Lyme disease by enzyme-linked immunosorbent assay with a peptide based on an immunodominant conserved region of *Borrelia burgdorferi* vlsE. J Clin Microbiol 1999;37(12):3990–6.

21. Boost MV, O'Donoghue MM, James A. Prevalence of *Staphylococcus aureus* carriage among dogs and their owners. Epidemiol Infect 2008;136(7):953–64.

22. Weese JS, Dick H, Willey BM, et al. Suspected transmission of methicillin-resistant *Staphylococcus aureus* between domestic pets and humans in veterinary clinics and in the household. Vet Microbiol 2006;115(1–3):148–55.

23. Demma LJ, Traeger MS, Nicholson WL, et al. Rocky Mountain spotted fever from an unexpected tick vector in Arizona. N Engl J Med 2005;353(6):587–94.

24. Demma LJ, Traeger M, Blau D, et al. Serologic evidence for exposure to *Rickettsia rickettsii* in eastern Arizona and recent emergence of Rocky Mountain spotted fever in this region. Vector Borne Zoonotic Dis 2006;6(4):423–9.

25. Demma LJ, Eremeeva M, Nicholson WL, et al. An outbreak of Rocky Mountain spotted fever associated with a novel tick vector, *Rhipicephalus sanguineus*, in Arizona, 2004: preliminary report. Ann N Y Acad Sci 2006;1078:342–3.

26. Nicholson WL, Gordon R, Demma LJ, et al. Spotted fever group rickettsial infection in dogs from eastern Arizona: how long has it been there? Ann N Y Acad Sci 2006;1078:519–22.

27. La SB, Raoult D. Laboratory diagnosis of rickettsioses: current approaches to diagnosis of old and new rickettsial diseases. J Clin Microbiol 1997;35(11):2715–27.

28. Espejo E, Alegre MD, Font B, et al. Antibodies to *Rickettsia conorii* in dogs: seasonal differences. Eur J Epidemiol 1993;9(3):344–6.

29. Greene CE, Marks MA, Lappin MR, et al. Comparison of latex agglutination, indirect immunofluorescent antibody, and enzyme immunoassay methods for serodiagnosis of Rocky Mountain spotted fever in dogs. Am J Vet Res 1993;54(1):20–8.

30. Dumler JS, Barbet AF, Bekker CP, et al. Reorganization of genera in the families Rickettsiaceae and Anaplasmataceae in the order Rckettsiales: unification of

some species of *Ehrlichia* with *Anaplasma, Cowdria* with *Ehrlichia* and *Ehrlichia* with *Neorickettsia*, descriptions of six new species combinations and designation of *Ehrlichia equi* and 'HGE agent' as subjective synonyms of *Ehrlichia phagocytophila*. Int J Syst Evol Microbiol 2001;51(Pt 6):2145–65.

31. Walker JS, Rundquist JD, Taylor R, et al. Clinical and clinicopathologic findings in tropical canine pancytopenia. J Am Vet Med Assoc 1970;157(1):43–55.
32. Maeda K, Markowitz N, Hawley RC, et al. Human infection with *Ehrlichia canis*, a leukocytic rickettsia. N Engl J Med 1987;316(14):853–6.
33. Anderson BE, Dawson JE, Jones DC, et al. *Ehrlichia chaffeensis*, a new species associated with human ehrlichiosis. J Clin Microbiol 1991;29(12):2838–42.
34. Murphy GL, Ewing SA, Whitworth LC, et al. A molecular and serologic survey of *Ehrlichia canis, E. chaffeensis*, and *E. ewingii* in dogs and ticks from Oklahoma. Vet Parasitol 1998;79(4):325–39.
35. Perez M, Bodor M, Zhang C, et al. Human infection with *Ehrlichia canis* accompanied by clinical signs in Venezuela. Ann N Y Acad Sci 2006;1078:110–7.
36. Anderson BE, Greene CE, Jones DC, et al. *Ehrlichia ewingii* sp. nov., the etiologic agent of canine granulocytic ehrlichiosis. Int J Syst Bacteriol 1992;42(2):299–302.
37. Buller RS, Arens M, Hmiel SP, et al. *Ehrlichia ewingii*, a newly recognized agent of human ehrlichiosis. N Engl J Med 1999;341(3):148–55.
38. Ewing SA, Roberson WR, Buckner RG, et al. A new strain of *Ehrlichia canis*. J Am Vet Med Assoc 1971;159(12):1771–4.
39. Bakken JS, Dumler JS, Chen SM, et al. Human granulocytic ehrlichiosis in the upper midwest United States. A new species emerging? J Am Med Assoc 1994;272(3):212–8.
40. Barlough JE, Rikihisa Y, Madigan JE, et al. Nested polymerase chain reaction for detection of *Ehrlichia risticii* genomic DNA in infected horses. Vet Parasitol 1997; 68(4):367–73.
41. Engvall EO, Pettersson B, Persson M, et al. A 16S rRNA-based PCR assay for detection and identification of granulocytic *Ehrlichia* species in dogs, horses, and cattle. J Clin Microbiol 1996;34(9):2170–4.
42. Walls JJ, Asanovich KM, Bakken JS, et al. Serologic evidence of a natural infection of white-tailed deer with the agent of human granulocytic ehrlichiosis in Wisconsin and Maryland. Clin Diagn Lab Immunol 1998;5(6):762–5.
43. Lappin MR, Breitschwerdt EB, Jensen WA, et al. Molecular and serologic evidence of *Anaplasma phagocytophilum* infection in cats in North America. J Am Vet Med Assoc 2004;225(6):893–6, 879.
44. Daniels TJ, Boccia TM, Varde S, et al. Geographic risk for Lyme disease and human granulocytic ehrlichiosis in southern New York State. Appl Environ Microbiol 1998;64(12):4663–9.
45. Schauber EM, Gertz SJ, Maple WT, et al. Coinfection of blacklegged ticks (Acari: Ixodidae) in Dutchess County, New York, with the agents of Lyme disease and human granulocytic ehrlichiosis. J Med Entomol 1998;35(5):901–3.
46. Belongia EA. Epidemiology and impact of coinfections acquired from *Ixodes* ticks. Vector Borne Zoonotic Dis 2002;2(4):265–73.
47. Swanson SJ, Neitzel D, Reed KD, et al. Coinfections acquired from *Ixodes* ticks. Clin Microbiol Rev 2006;19(4):708–27.
48. Paddock CD, Childs JE. *Ehrlichia chaffeensis*: a prototypical emerging pathogen. Clin Microbiol Rev 2003;16(1):37–64.
49. Paddock CD, Folk SM, Shore GM, et al. Infections with *Ehrlichia chaffeensis* and *Ehrlichia ewingii* in persons coinfected with human immunodeficiency virus. Clin Infect Dis 2001;33(9):1586–94.

50. Aguero-Rosenfeld ME, Horowitz HW, Wormser GP, et al. Human granulocytic ehrlichiosis: a case series from a medical center in New York state. Ann Intern Med 1996;125(11):904–8.

51. Bakken JS, Dumler JS. Clinical diagnosis and treatment of human granulocytotropic anaplasmosis. Ann N Y Acad Sci 2006;1078:236–47.

52. Suksawat J, Hegarty BC, Breitschwerdt EB, et al. Seroprevalence of *Ehrlichia canis, Ehrlichia equi*, and *Ehrlichia risticii* in sick dogs from North Carolina and Virginia. J Vet Intern Med 2000;14(1):50–5.

53. Comer JA, Nicholson WL, Olson JG, et al. Serologic testing for human granulocytic ehrlichiosis at a national referral center. J Clin Microbiol 1999;37(3):558–64.

54. Centers for disease control and prevention. Biological and chemical terrorism: strategic plan for preparedness and response. Recommendations of the CDC strategic planning workgroup. MMWR Recomm Rep 2000;49(RR–4):1–14.

55. Meinkoth KR, Morton RJ, Meinkoth JH. Naturally occurring tularemia in a dog. J Am Vet Med Assoc 2004;225(4):545–7, 538.

56. Gliatto JM, Rae JF, McDonough PL, et al. Feline tularemia on Nantucket island, Massachusetts. J Vet Diagn Invest 1994;6(1):102–5.

57. Baldwin CJ, Panciera RJ, Morton RJ, et al. Acute tularemia in three domestic cats. J Am Vet Med Assoc 1991;199(11):1602–5.

58. Liles WC, Burger RJ. Tularemia from domestic cats. West J Med 1993;158(6): 619–22.

59. Capellan J, Fong IW. Tularemia from a cat bite: case report and review of feline-associated tularemia. Clin Infect Dis 1993;16(4):472–5.

60. Podsiadly E, Chmielewski T, Sochon E, et al. *Bartonella henselae* in *Ixodes ricinus* ticks removed from dogs. Vector Borne Zoonotic Dis 2007;7(2):189–92.

61. Chang CC, Chomel BB, Kasten RW, et al. Molecular evidence of *Bartonella* spp. in questing adult *Ixodes pacificus* ticks in California. J Clin Microbiol 2001;39(4):1221–6.

62. Wikswo ME, Hu R, Metzger ME, et al. Detection of *Rickettsia rickettsii* and *Bartonella henselae* in *Rhipicephalus sanguineus* ticks from California. J Med Entomol 2007;44(1):158–62.

63. Billeter SA, Levy MG, Chomel BB, et al. Vector transmission of *Bartonella* species with emphasis on the potential for tick transmission. Med Vet Entomol 2008;22(1): 1–15.

64. Roux V, Eykyn SJ, Wyllie S, et al. *Bartonella vinsonii* subsp. *berkhoffii* as an agent of afebrile blood culture-negative endocarditis in a human. J Clin Microbiol 2000; 38(4):1698–700.

65. MacDonald KA, Chomel BB, Kittleson MD, et al. A prospective study of canine infective endocarditis in northern California (1999–2001): emergence of *Bartonella* as a prevalent etiologic agent. J Vet Intern Med 2004;18(1):56–64.

66. Welch DF, Carroll KC, Hofmeister EK, et al. Isolation of a new subspecies, *Bartonella vinsonii* subsp. *arupensis*, from a cattle rancher: identity with isolates found in conjunction with *Borrelia burgdorferi* and *Babesia microti* among naturally infected mice. J Clin Microbiol 1999;37(8):2598–601.

67. Pappalardo BL, Correa MT, York CC, et al. Epidemiologic evaluation of the risk factors associated with exposure and seroreactivity to *Bartonella vinsonii* in dogs. Am J Vet Res 1997;58(5):467–71.

68. Breitschwerdt EB, Hegarty BC, Hancock SI. Sequential evaluation of dogs naturally infected with *Ehrlichia canis, Ehrlichia chaffeensis, Ehrlichia equi, Ehrlichia ewingii*, or *Bartonella vinsonii*. J Clin Microbiol 1998;36(9):2645–51.

69. Baneth G, Breitschwerdt EB, Hegarty BC, et al. A survey of tick-borne bacteria and protozoa in naturally exposed dogs from Israel. Vet Parasitol 1998;74(2–4):133–42.

70. Chang CC, Kasten RW, Chomel BB, et al. Coyotes (*Canis latrans*) as the reservoir for a human pathogenic *Bartonella* sp: molecular epidemiology of *Bartonella vinsonii* subsp. *berkhoffii* infection in coyotes from central coastal California. J Clin Microbiol 2000;38(11):4193–200.

71. Suksawat J, Xuejie Y, Hancock SI, et al. Serologic and molecular evidence of coinfection with multiple vector-borne pathogens in dogs from Thailand. J Vet Intern Med 2001;15(5):453–62.

72. Masters EJ, Grigery CN, Masters RW. STARI, or Master's disease: lone star tick-vectored Lyme-like illness. Infect Dis Clin North Am 2008;22(2):361–76.

73. Masters EJ, Donnell HD. Lyme and/or lyme-like disease in Missouri. Mol Med 1995;92(7):346–53.

74. Campbell GL, Paul WS, Schriefer ME, et al. Epidemiologic and diagnostic studies of patients with suspected early Lyme disease, Missouri, 1990–1993. J Infect Dis 1995;172(2):470–80.

75. Varela AS, Luttrell MP, Howerth EW, et al. First culture isolation of *Borrelia lonestari*, putative agent of southern tick-associated rash illness. J Clin Microbiol 2004;42(3):1163–9.

76. Wormser GP, Masters E, Liveris D, et al. Microbiologic evaluation of patients from Missouri with erythema migrans. Clin Infect Dis 2005;40(3):423–8.

77. Philipp MT, Masters E, Wormser GP, et al. Serologic evaluation of patients from Missouri with erythema migrans-like skin lesions with the C6 Lyme test. Clin Vaccine Immunol 2006;13(10):1170–1.

78. Moyer PL, Varela AS, Luttrell MP, et al. White-tailed deer (Odocoileus virginianus) develop spirochetemia following experimental infection with *Borrelia lonestari*. Vet Microbiol 2006;115(1–3):229–36.

79. Moore VA, Varela AS, Yabsley MJ, et al. Detection of *Borrelia lonestari*, putative agent of southern tick-associated rash illness, in white-tailed deer (*Odocoileus virginianus*) from the southeastern United States. J Clin Microbiol 2003;41(1): 424–7.

80. Kjemtrup AM, Kocan AA, Whitworth L, et al. There are at least three genetically distinct small piroplasms from dogs. Int J Parasitol 2000;30(14):1501–5.

81. Kjemtrup AM, Wainwright K, Miller M, et al. *Babesia conradae*, sp. nov., a small canine *Babesia* identified in California. Vet Parasitol 2006;138(1–2):103–11.

82. Irizarry-Rovira AR, Stephens J, Christian J, et al. *Babesia gibsoni* infection in a dog from Indiana. Vet Clin Pathol 2001;30(4):180–8.

83. Macintire DK, Boudreaux MK, West GD, et al. *Babesia gibsoni* infection among dogs in the southeastern United States. J Am Vet Med Assoc 2002;220(3):325–9.

84. Conrad PA, Kjemtrup AM, Carreno RA, et al. Description of *Babesia duncani* n.sp. (Apicomplexa: Babesiidae) from humans and its differentiation from other piroplasms. Int J Parasitol 2006;36(7):779–89.

85. Dryden M, Payne P, McBride A, et al. Efficacy of fipronil (9.8% w/w) + (S)-methoprene (8.8% w/w) and imidacloprid (8.8% w/w) + permethrin (44% w/w) against *Dermacentor variabilis* (American dog tick) on dogs. Vet Ther 2008;9(1):15–25.

86. Dryden MW, Payne PA, Smith V, et al. Evaluation of an imidacloprid (8.8% w/w)–permethrin (44.0% w/w) topical spot-on and a fipronil (9.8% w/w)–(S)-methoprene (8.8% w/w) topical spot-on to repel, prevent attachment, and kill adult *Rhipicephalus sanguineus* and *Dermacentor variabilis* ticks on dogs. Vet Ther 2006;7(3):187–98.

87. Dryden MW, Payne PA, Smith V, et al. Efficacy of imidacloprid (8.8% w/w) plus permethrin (44% w/w) spot-on topical solution against *Amblyomma americanum* infesting dogs using a natural tick exposure model. Vet Ther 2006;7(2):99–106.

88. Estrada-Pena A, Ascher F. Comparison of an amitraz-impregnated collar with topical administration of fipronil for prevention of experimental and natural infestations by the brown dog tick (*Rhipicephalus sanguineus*). J Am Vet Med Assoc 1999;214(12):1799–803.

89. Jernigan AD, McTier TL, Chieffo C, et al. Efficacy of selamectin against experimentally induced tick (*Rhipicephalus sanguineus* and *Dermacentor variabilis*) infestations on dogs. Vet Parasitol 2000;91(3–4):359–75.

90. Bishop BF, Bruce CI, Evans NA, et al. Selamectin: a novel broad-spectrum endectocide for dogs and cats. Vet Parasitol 2000;91(3–4):163–76.

91. Chu HJ, Chavez LG Jr, Blumer BM, et al. Immunogenicity and efficacy study of a commercial *Borrelia burgdorferi* bacterin. J Am Vet Med Assoc 1992;201(3):403–11.

92. Levy SA. Use of a C6 ELISA test to evaluate the efficacy of a whole-cell bacterin for the prevention of naturally transmitted canine *Borrelia burgdorferi* infection. Vet Ther 2002;3(4):420–4.

93. de Silva AM, Telford SR3, Brunet LR, et al. *Borrelia burgdorferi* OspA is an arthropod-specific transmission-blocking Lyme disease vaccine. J Exp Med 1996;183(1):271–5.

94. Piesman J, Dolan MC. Protection against Lyme disease spirochete transmission provided by prompt removal of nymphal *Ixodes scapularis* (Acari: Ixodidae). J Med Entomol 2002;39(3):509–12.

95. Nadelman RB, Nowakowski J, Fish D, et al. Prophylaxis with single-dose doxycycline for the prevention of Lyme disease after an *Ixodes scapularis* tick bite. N Engl J Med 2001;345(2):79–84.

Pets and Antimicrobial Resistance

Jamie K. Umber, DVM, Jeff B. Bender, DVM, MS*

KEYWORDS

- MRSA • Multidrug-resistant *Salmonella*
- Nosocomial infections • Antimicrobial resistance

The public has become aware of so-called "super bugs" such as methicillin-resistant *Staphylococcus aureus* (MRSA), extensively drug-resistant tuberculosis, and hypervirulent *Clostridium difficile* through the popular media and personal anecdotes of friends and family members. These organisms often are linked to greater disease severity, longer hospitalization, and increased care and treatment costs in human patients. They also highlight the interconnectedness of human and animal health, because resistant micro-organisms can afflict both humans and animals. The use of antimicrobial agents in veterinary medicine is suspected of being an important factor in the development of antimicrobial-resistant organisms in humans. The emergence of drug-resistant food-borne pathogens such as *Salmonella*, *Campylobacter*, and *Escherichia coli* are of particular concern. This evolving challenge to human and animal health has no quick solutions. Health professionals realize that antimicrobial resistance is a multifaceted problem and that the solutions will require active efforts by practitioners of both human and veterinary medicine. This article reviews current antimicrobial-resistant organisms and the reasons for their emergence to explain the spread of resistance and to summarize methods for control. The focus is on the emergence of antimicrobial-resistant organisms isolated from companion animals (ie, dogs, cats, and "pocket pets") and the subsequent implications for public health.

HOW RESISTANCE DEVELOPS

Antimicrobial resistance may develop by several different mechanisms that vary depending on the organism and the class of antimicrobial agent involved. Mechanisms for bacterial resistance often are categorized as either intrinsic or acquired (**Table 1**). Intrinsic resistance (sometimes called "natural resistance") mechanisms are those specified by naturally occurring genes found in the host organism's DNA. Acquired resistance mechanisms involve the development or acquisition of genes that encode antimicrobial resistance. This process occurs through mutations of genetic material, the transfer of genetic material between organisms, or both. For

University of Minnesota, 136F ABLMS, 1354 Eckles Avenue, St. Paul, MN 55108, USA
* Corresponding author.
E-mail address: bende002@umn.edu (J.B. Bender).

Vet Clin Small Anim 39 (2009) 279–292
doi:10.1016/j.cvsm.2008.10.016
0195-5616/08/$ – see front matter © 2009 Elsevier Inc. All rights reserved.

vetsmall.theclinics.com

Table 1
Common mechanisms by which antimicrobial resistance can develop

Category	Mechanism
Intrinsic	Organism lacks target sites of antimicrobial (eg, organism may lack a cell wall)
	Organism lacks transport mechanisms that allow the antimicrobial to be effective
Acquired	Mutation of DNA
	Transfer of chromosomal DNA
	Transfer of extra-chromosomal DNA (ie, on plasmids, bacteriophages, transposons, and other mobile genetic material)

example, genes that encode for resistance determinants can be transferred between organisms on plasmids, bacteriophages, transposons, and other mobile genetic material.[1] Occasionally, broad resistance can be transferred so that organisms become resistant to an entire class of antimicrobials (eg, macrolides).[2]

A number of driving forces can increase the development of resistance. These contributors include the use of antimicrobial agents at concentrations close to or below the minimum inhibitory concentration for particular organisms, the overuse of antimicrobial agents, and the use of broad-spectrum antimicrobial agents. The use of antimicrobial agents at inappropriate doses and the overuse of antimicrobial agents can create selective pressure within the host or the environment, fostering the development of resistant organisms. The use of broad-spectrum antimicrobial agents can affect an array of organisms, with some—including some organisms that were not the intended target of the treatment—acquiring resistance. Situations that allow the transfer of resistance between organisms, such as close physical contact, or environmental factors that allow the growth or persistence of infective organisms, such as improper cleaning/disinfection practices, also can increase the development of resistance.

Factors that favor the acquisition of antimicrobial-resistant infections include hospitalization, the use of invasive medical devices or invasive procedures, and immune system compromise. Longer duration of hospital stay can be associated with more exposure events; the use of invasive devices and/or procedures circumvents the body's natural defense systems; and immunocompromised patients are more susceptible to opportunistic infections. Of particular concern are multidrug-resistant (MDR) organisms, that is, organisms that are resistant to one or more classes of antimicrobial agents.

IMPORTANT ANTIMICROBIAL-RESISTANT PATHOGENS

In 1941 the "miracle drug" penicillin was introduced. Within 2 years drug resistance to penicillin was documented. Since then, many drug-resistant human pathogens have emerged, such as *Mycobacterium tuberculosis, Staphylococcus aureus, Neisseria gonorrhoeae* (gonorrhea), and *Plasmodium falciparum* (malaria). Similar situations of drug-specific resistance and drug-resistant organisms in veterinary medicine have been documented that affect treatment outcomes, length of care, and costs. Examples include resistant *Staphylococcus intermedius* from skin lesions, fluoroquinolone-resistant *E. coli* isolated from urinary tract infections, and nosocomial pathogens (such as *Enterococcus, Acinetobacter, Klebsiella*, and MRSA).[3–8] Unfortunately, there are limited data in the veterinary realm regarding the mechanisms of transmission of resistance elements, the impact of antimicrobial resistance, or an evaluation of control strategies. This situation will change with the developing field of veterinary infection control.

It often is assumed that the use of antimicrobials in food animals is a significant culprit in the development of antimicrobial resistance in humans because of the potential transfer of resistant bacteria via food. Some authors, however, have suggested that the role of food animals in the transmission of antimicrobial resistance may be over-emphasized in the scientific literature.[9,10] Pets, especially cats and dogs, are potential sources of spread of antimicrobial resistance because of the common use of antimicrobial agents in these animals and their close contact with humans.[9] In 2002, companion or nonfood animals accounted for 37% of the animal health pharmaceutical products sales in the European Union, with pets often receiving medically important antimicrobial agents such as cephalosporins or fluoroquinolones.[9] Of the fluoroquinolones and cephalosporins used in all animals in Denmark in 2003, 45% of the fluoroquinolones and 55% of the cephalosporins were used in companion animals.[11,12] This amount is concerning when one considers that there are 1.2 million dogs and cats in Denmark—a small population of animals compared with the population of food animals (23 million slaughter pigs, 130 million broiler chickens, and 1.2 million cattle).[11] It is possible a similar situation exists in the United States, although statistics for antimicrobial use are not available.

MULTIDRUG-RESISTANT *SALMONELLA* INFECTIONS

Some recent examples highlight the impact of antimicrobial resistance on the clinical outcomes of veterinary patients and the spread of resistant organisms to and from human caretakers. These examples include the recent identification of MDR *Salmonella* Typhimurium from dogs, cats, and pocket pets (eg, hamsters, mice, and rats).[13,14]

In Minnesota, as part of an integrated human–animal surveillance program, *S.* Typhimurium isolates from veterinary diagnostic samples are forwarded to the Minnesota Department of Health for molecular subtyping and antimicrobial susceptibility testing. In December 1999, five *S.* Typhimurium isolates from cats had the same pulsed-field gel electrophoresis (PFGE) pattern. These isolates were resistant to ampicillin, chloramphenicol, streptomycin, sulfamethoxazole, and tetracycline (R-type ACSSuT). Upon investigating, it was found that all the samples were submitted from a regional humane society. Seven human cases were documented among individuals who had recently adopted kittens from the shelter or who had come in contact with a person that had recently adopted a kitten. A number of kittens were diagnosed with and died from salmonellosis. This case provides evidence of both zoonotic transmission to staff and spread to other animals in the shelter. Of concern, most of the human cases were in children (median age, 6 years). The median duration of illness was 8 days (range, 5–11 days). All seven identified human patients had sought medical care; one child was hospitalized.[14] The costs of cleaning, disinfection, loss of income, and employee training were substantial. Similar costly nosocomial events have occurred in equine veterinary clinics.[15]

Pet food and treats also can serve as a vehicle for animal and human *Salmonella* infections. In 2006 and 2007, 70 human cases of *S.* Schwarzengrund were found to be associated with contaminated dry dog food.[16] In 2002, MDR human infections with *Salmonella* Newport were reported among five patients who handled commercial pet treats in Calgary, Alberta, Canada.[17] Before this outbreak, *Salmonella* had been identified frequently from pet treats made from pig ears.[18] In a United States study, 28 *Salmonella* isolates from pet treats (36%) were resistant to at least one antimicrobial agent, and 10 (13%) isolates displayed resistance to four or more antimicrobial agents.[19] These human outbreaks and isolation of *Salmonella* from pet treats and pet food often do not correspond to documented or reported pet illnesses, representing either asymptomatic carriage, the lack of a sensitive veterinary surveillance network to detect these outbreaks in pets, or both.

Outbreaks associated with pocket pets also have been documented recently.[13] In 2004, *Salmonella* Typhimurium was cultured from hamsters from a regional pet distributor. Human cases (n = 28) linked to this rodent-associated strain were primarily in children. Of 22 patients, 13 (59%) reported exposure to pet hamsters, mice, or rats. Human, rodent, and environmental isolates were resistant to multiple drugs. The authors postulated that pet rodents probably are an underrecognized source of human *Salmonella* infection.

METHICILLIN-RESISTANT *STAPHYLOCOCCUS AUREUS*

Staphylococcus aureus has long been recognized as an important human pathogen and is the leading cause of suppurative infections in humans. These infections include superficial skin infections such as boils and furuncles and more invasive infections such as bloodstream infections, pneumonia, osteomyelitis, and endocarditis. *S. aureus* also is a major cause of nosocomial infections, including surgical site infections and infections associated with indwelling medical devices. Penicillinase-producing strains of *S. aureus* initially were rare, but now most *S. aureus* strains produce penicillinases. Methicillin was introduced in 1961, and resistance was reported within a year.[20] Methicillin resistance now serves as a marker for resistance to β-lactam antimicrobials. Currently in some United States hospitals, 55% or more of *S. aureus* isolates are methicillin resistant.[21] Established risk factors for MRSA in humans include current or recent hospitalization or surgery, residence in a long-term care facility, dialysis, and indwelling percutaneous medical devices and catheters.[22,23] Recently, community-associated cases not linked to traditional sources of MRSA infection have been recognized also.[24]

MRSA infections are being reported increasingly in dogs, horses, pigs, and cats.[25–28] The potential for MRSA transmission from pets to humans is unknown and requires further assessment. Several case studies have documented the occurrence of MRSA among family members and their asymptomatic household pets.[29–31] These case reports have suggested that the success of human treatment involved the identification and treatment of the household pet. This suggestion probably is true for human households where there is evidence of ongoing or recurrent infection among human family members. Preliminary evidence suggests that dogs and cats are colonized transiently, likely carrying MRSA for several weeks (Jeff Bender DVM, unpublished data). The implication is that antimicrobial treatment of the asymptomatic pet in a household is not needed unless there is evidence of ongoing or recurrent human infection(s).

Symptomatic MRSA illness has been documented in companion animals as well.[32] In a review of animals presented to the University of Minnesota Veterinary Medical Center (VMC) with MRSA, most had nonhealing skin lesions. Most isolates from these animals were genotype USA100 and were indistinguishable from strains associated with human health care. Interviews of owners revealed that at least one member of each of the families who owned infected pets had been hospitalized recently, had ongoing severe illness (eg, was undergoing chemotherapy), or was a health care provider. These data suggest that the pet infections probably were acquired from their owners. This supposition is supported by detection of MRSA in asymptomatic pets that reside in long-term care facilities.[33]

These MRSA situations highlight the need for owner education about potential risks, precautions, and hand hygiene. As part of client education at the University of

Minnesota VMC, staff inform owners of MRSA patients of the potential risks to themselves and other family members, provide fact sheets and verbal consultations on pet care and handling, and encourage the pet owner to consult with their physician. Evidence of this traditionally human pathogen in pets requires improvements in infection-control efforts at veterinary clinics/hospitals. Extra precautions implemented at the VMC include staff notification, prompt cluster evaluations, clinician alerts in electronic patient medical records, in-service education and review of hand hygiene, and enhanced isolation procedures. MRSA strains also have been recovered from environmental surfaces in the VMC clinic, prompting greater attention to patient placement and disinfection protocols.

Concerns about MDR staphylococcal organisms are not restricted to MRSA. From 2001 through 2005, the University of Tennessee has documented an increase in the amount of oxacillin resistance among *S. intermedius* strains.[34] Jones and colleagues[34] observed that one in five *Staphylococcus* spp isolates was oxacillin resistant. In addition, *S. schleiferi* is inherently oxacillin resistant and commonly is isolated from healthy dogs and dogs with otitis and pyoderma.[35] Transfer of resistant *S. intermedius* organisms between dogs and their owners has been observed.[3] This observation raises the possibility that resistance genes might be transferred between different bacterial species (ie, transfer of resistance elements between *S. intermedius* and *S. aureus)* and reinforces ongoing concerns about the overuse of antimicrobial agents in pets and the potential transfer of resistant organisms to human caretakers.[3]

NOSOCOMIAL INFECTIONS

Nosocomial (ie, hospital-associated) infections have been recognized increasingly in veterinary hospitals. As in human nosocomial infections, the most commonly identified pathogens associated with veterinary nosocomial infections are Gram-positive cocci (eg, staphylococci and enterococci), members of the Enterobacteriaceae family, and non-fermentative Gram-negative bacilli (eg, *Acinetobacter* and *Pseudomonas*).[36,37] Nosocomial organisms often are resistant to antimicrobial agents.[38]

Several studies have identified nosocomial infections (some involving outbreaks) in dogs and cats with *Acinetobacter* spp, *Clostridium perfringens, Enterococcus* spp, *E. coli, Klebsiella* spp, *Pseudomonas* spp, *Serratia marcescens,* and *Staphylococcus* spp (eg, MRSA) **(Table 2)**.[5,8,39–45] *Salmonella* spp were identified in most of the outbreaks in small animal facilities that had evidence of both nosocomial spread and zoonotic infections. Nosocomial infections often are associated with bloodstream infections, urinary tract infections, respiratory tract infections (eg, pneumonia), surgical wound infections, and/or infectious diarrhea.[38] In two studies, postoperative surgical wounds were the most common site of infection in pets.[5,46] Murtaugh and Mason[46] found that postoperative surgical wounds accounted for 46% of known nosocomial infections.

Factors linked to nosocomial infections in human health care facilities also are common in veterinary hospitals. These factors include the use of invasive devices (eg, intravenous and urinary catheters, surgical instruments), implantation of orthopedic hardware, longer hospitalization stays, induced immunosuppression with chemotherapies, and the use of antimicrobial agents. In one study, an increased duration of stay in the small animal ICU was associated with positive catheter-tip cultures and nosocomial urinary tract infections.[47]

The probability of a patient developing a nosocomial infection depends on many factors. These factors include the virulence of the agent, the susceptibility of the patient to that particular agent, the amount and route of exposure, the number and

Table 2
Reported nosocomial events in small animal facilities in the United States and Canada, 1975–2007

Organism	MDR	Year	Number and Species Involved	Zoonotic Transmission (Yes/No)	Type of Facility	Reference
Klebsiella spp	yes	1977–1978	23 dogs 1 cat	NA	Veterinary teaching hospital	5
Salmonella travis	NA	1978–1979	17 dogs	NA	Veterinary teaching hospital	42
Serratia marcescens	yes	NA	81 dogs and cats	NA	Veterinary clinic	41
Salmonella krefeld	NA	1984	20 dogs	yes	Veterinary teaching hospital	43
Clostridium perfringens	NA	1985–1988	30 dogs	NA	Veterinary teaching hospital	39
Salmonella Typhimurium	yes	1999	12 cats	yes	Veterinary clinic	14
S. Typhimurium	yes	1999	Kittens	yes	Veterinary clinic	14
Acinetobacter baumannii	yes	1998–2000	10 dogs 5 cats (1 horse)	NA	Veterinary teaching hospital	8
Escherichia coli	yes	1998–2000	19 dogs	NA	Veterinary teaching hospital	45
S. Typhimurium	yes	2000	3 dogs 4 cats	yes	Veterinary clinic	14
S. Typhimurium	yes	1999–2000	9 kittens	yes	Animal shelter	14
Clostridium difficile	no	2002	48 dogs	NA	Veterinary teaching hospital	44
Escherichia coli	yes	2003	6 dogs	NA	Veterinary teaching hospital	4
Staphylococcus aureus (MRSA)	yes	2007	4 dogs 2 cats	NA	Veterinary teaching hospital	6

Abbreviation: NA, not available.

type of invasive procedures that the patient undergoes, and prior antimicrobial therapy.[37] Organisms that cause nosocomial infections may be intrinsically pathogenic, or they may be part of the normal flora of the patient (eg, on the skin, in the upper respiratory tract, or in the gastrointestinal tract).[38] The use of antimicrobials can alter a patient's bacterial flora by diminishing susceptible bacteria and allowing resistant bacteria to flourish.[46,48] This alteration, together with the existence of fomites (eg, keyboards, stethoscopes, thermometers, and other devices) and personnel that can harbor resistant bacteria, often leads to the promotion and propagation of antimicrobial resistance in nosocomial pathogens, particularly to the antimicrobials most frequently used in that particular hospital.[38] At the University of Minnesota VMC, MDR E. coli was isolated more commonly from patients in the ICU than from patients seen as VMC outpatients on the community practice service (**Table 3**). This difference probably reflected antimicrobial use in the ICU and highlights the need to take precautions to prevent nosocomial spread of pathogens, especially among high-risk patients.

Many veterinary hospitals have instituted programs attempting to prevent and control nosocomial infections. These efforts include improving hand hygiene and the cleaning and disinfection of facilities and equipment, implementation of policies for patient isolation, establishment of an antimicrobial use committee, restriction of antimicrobial use, and implementation of microbiologic surveillance systems (**Fig. 1**).[46] Surveillance is important for establishing baseline rates of infection. For example, a review of 663 tibial plateau–leveling osteotomy (TPLO) surgeries at the University of Minnesota VMC identified surgical site infections in 23 patients (3.6%). These baseline data provided a means to summarize key pathogens, surgeon-specific infection rates, overall rates of infection, and success of implemented intervention programs.[49]

STEPS TO PREVENT DEVELOPMENT OF ANTIMICROBIAL RESISTANCE

The increase in MDR infections in animals and humans demonstrates the need to develop and implement measures to monitor and control the spread of antimicrobial resistance among companion animals. These measures should be tailored to individual hospitals or clinics but generally should include guidelines for appropriate antimicrobial use and infection-control policies.

A number of guidelines regarding antimicrobial use have been produced by the federal government (eg, the Centers for Disease Control and Prevention, the Food and Drug Administration, and the United States Department of Agriculture), by advocacy groups, and by professional organizations (eg, the American Veterinary Medical Association [AVMA]). The AVMA issued guidelines for antimicrobial use in its "Judicious Therapeutic Use of Antimicrobials" policy.[50] Several species-specific (ie, swine, feline/canine, bovine, and poultry) policies are available on the AVMA Web site. The dog and

Source	Number of Isolates	Pansensitive[a] n (%)	MDR[b] n (%)
Community practice	102	70 (69)	4 (4)
ICU	113	42 (37)	42 (37)

Table 3
Antimicrobial susceptibility of fecal E. coli isolates from outpatient community practice and inpatient ICU patients at the University of Minnesota Veterinary Medical Center, 2005

Katherine Peterson, DVM and Jeff B. Bender, DVM, MS, unpublished data, 2005.
[a] Sensitive to all antimicrobial agents on the panel; chi-square = 21.3; P<.01.
[b] Chi-square = 35.2; P<.01.

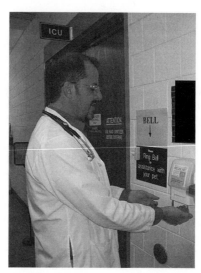

Fig. 1. Convenient placement of hand-sanitizers improves hand hygiene compliance.

cat recommendations were adapted from the AVMA's original guidelines (**Box 1**).[51] The position statement of these guidelines states "Once the decision is reached to use antimicrobial therapy, veterinarians should strive to optimize therapeutic efficacy, minimize resistance to antimicrobial agents, and protect public and animal health."[50,51] Examples of judicious veterinary antimicrobial use include avoiding antimicrobial treatment in asymptomatic and/or unnecessary situations (such as viral infections, parasitism, or nutritional imbalances that will not respond to antimicrobial therapies).

Furthermore, education about antimicrobial resistance and awareness of judicious use guidelines need to be included in veterinary training. This training could involve the incorporation of practice guidelines to aid students and clinicians in making appropriate treatment decisions for a variety of common diseases. In human medicine, practice guidelines have been published for appropriate treatment of ear infections, sinusitis, and diarrhea.[52–54] These evidence-based recommendations create performance measures that have been shown to result in a change in behavior, such as decreased or more appropriate antimicrobial prescription.[55] To ensure success, these measures need to be accompanied by client education. For example, community-wide educational interventions directed at human health care providers and parents have been successful in reducing antimicrobial use for acute respiratory infections.[56,57] There are, however, several reasons for non-adherence to guidelines. Among these reasons are guidelines that are too long or contain too many recommendations, guidelines of varying quality (some based on randomized, controlled studies and some based only on expert opinion), and confusion created by guidelines on the same subject issued by different societies and with slightly different recommendations.[55]

Encouraging the appropriate use of antimicrobial agents in companion animals (eg, through guidelines) is necessary for multiple reasons. Compared with food animal medicine, antimicrobial use in companion animal medicine more closely mirrors antimicrobial use in human medicine and therefore may have a more significant impact on public health. For example, the transmission of antimicrobial resistance may be enhanced because virtually the same classes of antimicrobial agents are used in human medicine and in small animal practice.[9] Patient compliance and selective pressures also may be more of an issue in veterinary medicine than in human medicine

---

Box 1
Basic guidelines for judicious therapeutic use of antimicrobials

1. Emphasize preventive health care that decreases the likelihood of patients developing infections that would require antimicrobial treatment.

   Follow recommended preventive health protocols (eg, vaccination, parasite control) when possible and appropriate.

   Educate clients regarding proper husbandry and hygiene.

2. Limit antimicrobial use to appropriate clinical indications.

   Definitive diagnosis should be established whenever possible, and empiric use of antimicrobial agents should be avoided.

3. Consider therapeutic alternatives before using antimicrobial therapy.

4. Use culture and susceptibility results to aid in the appropriate selection of antimicrobial agents.

5. Use narrow-spectrum antimicrobial agents whenever appropriate.

6. Use antimicrobial agents considered important in treating refractory infections in human or veterinary medicine only after careful review and reasonable justification.

7. Treat for the shortest effective period possible to minimize therapeutic exposure to antimicrobial agents.

   Further testing (eg, culture and sensitivity, complete blood cell counts, urinalyses) at the conclusion of therapy may help determine if additional therapy is needed.

8. A valid veterinarian–client–patient relationship must exist for the judicious use of antimicrobial agents.

9. Prescribe extra-label antimicrobial therapy only in accordance with all federal laws.

10. Work with those responsible for the care of animals to ensure judicious use of antimicrobial agents (eg, appropriate and reliable dose application of the drug) and explain potential adverse reactions of prescribed antimicrobial agents and what to do if such reactions occur.

11. Optimize therapeutic antimicrobial regimens using current pharmacologic information and principles.

    Antimicrobial agents chosen should be effective against the targeted organism and should be able to penetrate the affected organ in a proper concentration.

12. When combination antimicrobial treatment is advantageous, avoid the use of drugs whose actions are antagonistic.

13. Do not use prophylactic antimicrobials as a substitute for good animal health management.

14. Minimize environmental contamination with antimicrobial agents whenever possible.

15. Maintain accurate records of treatment and outcome to evaluate therapeutic regimens.

16. Recognize risk factors for infections in cats and dogs and prevent or correct them whenever possible.

Data from American Veterinary Medical Association. AVMA policy—judicious therapeutic use of antimicrobials. Available at: http://www.avma.org/issues/policy/jtua.asp. Accessed May, 2008.

(consider "pilling" the adult cat versus an adult human). The results of at least one veterinary study suggest that the development of specific antimicrobial use guidelines for use in individual hospitals and clinics can have a positive effect on prudent antimicrobial use.[58]

In addition to guidelines for antimicrobial use, infection-control programs for veterinary hospitals/clinics are needed to help prevent the development of MDR pathogens and to control nosocomial infections. For infection-control programs to be most effective, personnel are needed to monitor infections and to ensure that appropriate policies are developed and followed. Infection-control programs and policies should include improved design of clinics and hospitals, the development of evidence-based policies, and the training of clinicians and other staff on judicious use guidelines, husbandry and hygiene, and environmental cleaning and disinfection. The recent publication, "*Compendium of Veterinary Standard Precautions: Zoonotic Disease Prevention in Veterinary Personnel*," provides guidelines for the protection of staff from zoonotic infections.[37] These guidelines can be applied broadly to protect patient health by promoting greater emphasis on patient precautions, hand hygiene, and surveillance. These measures are necessary when one considers the type of high-risk patients (eg, oncology or complicated surgical patients and neonates) being treated in veterinary clinics. These high-risk groups are more apt to acquire MDR nosocomial pathogens. As demonstrated previously, many veterinary patients may be exposed to or acquire these organisms within veterinary clinics or outside clinics from various environmental sources, animals, or humans.

Surveillance of MDR organisms is key to detecting novel organisms. An infection-control surveillance system should include dedicated personnel, funding, and laboratory support. To evaluate the success of a program, metrics should evaluate whether decreases in inappropriate antimicrobial use or increases in correct antimicrobial use occur. Future efforts to develop computer programs that can track antimicrobial use and periodically evaluate and record MDR organisms would be helpful to determine program success. The potential benefits of having a monitoring program include improving patient treatment and care and early detection of unusual resistance patterns.[59] At present the monitoring of antimicrobial-resistant organisms in companion animals is limited and may be done only in some (often larger or multisite) veterinary clinic settings. Most surveillance is done at veterinary teaching hospitals, which are inherently biased toward patients with severe or protracted illnesses. An additional challenge is that bacterial identification and testing for antimicrobial susceptibility are not always performed (for many possible reasons, but economic costs to clients often are cited as a main deterrent). This lack may lead to inappropriate empiric treatment (eg, antimicrobial treatment of uncomplicated viral infections).[9]

SUMMARY

The changing status of pets in society has allowed more and closer physical contact between humans and their pets (eg, through shared living spaces) and has created an opportunity for humans and pets to exchange micro-organisms. In addition, the use of antimicrobial agents increases selective pressure on micro-organisms so that microbial resistance can develop. This alone should encourage veterinarians to reevaluate antimicrobial treatment options for their patients. Antimicrobial treatment may affect not only veterinary patients but also pet owners and the larger community.

Although antimicrobials have significantly improved the ability to treat infectious diseases of bacterial origin, the development of new antimicrobials is no longer a top research and development priority.[60] Instead, there now is a long list of microbes that have become resistant to many different classes of drugs and therapeutic regimens.[1] Also, it is not only humans and animals that can serve to transmit micro-organisms and perpetuate resistance. The environment can serve as a reservoir for new (and old) resistance mechanisms, because many antimicrobial molecules can exist for years.[1,61] Client and professional education, pathogen surveillance, effective cleaning and disinfection, the use of appropriate bacterial culture and sensitivity techniques, and the creation of treatment guidelines will be important to achieve success in using antimicrobial agents appropriately.

REFERENCES

1. Alekshun MN, Levy SB. Molecular mechanisms of antibacterial multidrug resistance. Cellule 2007;128:1037–50.
2. Davison HC, Woolhouse MEJ, Low JC, et al. What is antibiotic resistance and how can we measure it? Trends Microbiol 2000;8(12):554–9.
3. Guardabassi L, Loeber ME, Jacobson A, et al. Transmission of multiple antimicrobial-resistant Staphylococcus intermedius between dogs affected by deep pyoderma and their owners. Vet Microbiol 2004;98:23–7.
4. Ogeer-Gyles J, Mathews K, Weese JS, et al. Evaluation of catheter-associated urinary tract infections and multi-drug-resistant Escherichia coli isolates from the urine of dogs with indwelling urinary catheters. J Am Vet Med Assoc 2006; 229(10):1584–9.
5. Glickman LT. Veterinary nosocomial (hospital-acquired) Klebsiella infections. J Am Vet Med Assoc 1981;179:1389–92.
6. Weese JS, Faires M, Rousseau J, et al. Cluster of methicillin-resistant Staphylococcus aureus colonization in a small animal intensive care unit. J Am Vet Med Assoc 2007;231(9):1361–4.
7. Ganiere J, Medaille C, Mangion C, et al. Antimicrobial drug susceptibility of Staphylococcus intermedius clinical isolates from canine pyoderma. J Vet Med B Infect Dis Vet Public Health 2005;52(1):25–31.
8. Boerlin P, Eugster S, Gaschen F, et al. Transmission of opportunistic pathogens in a veterinary teaching hospital. Vet Microbiol 2001;82(4):347–59.
9. Guardabassi L, Schwarz S, Lloyd DH, et al. Pet animals as reservoirs of antimicrobial-resistant bacteria. J Antimicrob Chemother 2004;54(2):321–32.
10. Barber DA, Miller GY, McNamara PE, et al. Models of antimicrobial resistance and foodborne illness: examining assumptions and practical applications. J Food Prot 2003;66(4):700–9.
11. Heuer OE, Jensen VF, Hammerum AM, et al. Antimicrobial drug consumption in companion animals. Emerg Infect Dis 2005;11:344–5.
12. DANMAP. Use of antimicrobial agents and occurrence of antimicrobial resistance in bacteria from food animals, foods and humans in Denmark. ISSN 2003; 1600–2032. Available at: http://www.danmap.org/pdfFiles/Danmap_2003.pdf. Accessed December, 2008.
13. Swanson SJ, Snider C, Braden CR, et al. Multidrug-resistant Salmonella enterica serotype Typhimurium associated with pet rodents. N Engl J Med 2007;356(1):21–8.
14. Wright JG, Tengelsen LA, Smith KE, et al. Multidrug-resistant Salmonella Typhimurium in four animal facilities. Emerg Infect Dis 2005;11(8):1235–41.
15. Dargatz DA, Traub-Dargatz JL. Multidrug-resistant Salmonella and nosocomial infections. Vet Clin North Am Equine Pract 2004;20(3):587–600.
16. Centers for Disease Control. Multistate outbreak of human Salmonella infections caused by contaminated dry dog food—United States, 2006–2007. MMWR Morb Mortal Wkly Rep 2008;57(19):521–4.
17. Pitout JD, Reisbig MD, Mulvey M, et al. Association between handling of pet treats and infection with Salmonella enterica serotype Newport expressing the AmpC beta-lactamase, CMY-2. J Clin Microbiol 2003;41(10):4578–82.

18. Clark C, Cunningham J, Ahmed R, et al. Characterization of *Salmonella* associated with pig ear dog treats in Canada. J Clin Microbiol 2001;39(11):3962–8.

19. White DG, Datta A, McDermott P, et al. Antimicrobial susceptibility and genetic relatedness of Salmonella serovars isolated from animal-derived dog treats in the USA. J Antimicrob Chemother 2003;52(5):860–3.

20. Chambers HF. The changing epidemiology of *Staphylococcus aureus*? Emerg Infect Dis 2001;7(2):178–82.

21. A report from the NNIS System. National Nosocomial Infections Surveillance (NNIS) System Report, data summary from January 1992 through June 2003, issued August 2003. Am J Infect Control 2003;31(8):481–98.

22. Brumfitt W, Hamilton-Miller J. Methicillin-resistant *Staphylococcus aureus*. N Engl J Med 1989;320:1188–96.

23. Lowy FD. *Staphylococcus aureus* infections. N Engl J Med 1998;339(8):520–32.

24. Naimi T, LeDell K, Boxrud D, et al. Epidemiology and clonality of community-acquired methicillin-resistant *Staphylococcus aureus* in Minnesota, 1996–1998. Clin Infect Dis 2001;33(7):990–6.

25. Bender JB, Torres SM, Gilbert SM, et al. Isolation of methicillin-resistant *Staphylococcus aureus* from a non-healing abscess in a cat. Vet Rec 2005;157(13): 388–9.

26. Baptiste KE, Williams K, Willams NJ, et al. Methicillin-resistant staphylococci in companion animals. Emerg Infect Dis 2005;11(12):1942–4.

27. Weese JS, Archambault M, Willey BM, et al. Methicillin-resistant *Staphylococcus aureus* in horses and horse personnel, 2000–2002. Emerg Infect Dis 2005;11(3): 430–5.

28. Armand-Lefevre L, Ruimy R, Andremont A, et al. Clonal comparison of *Staphylococcus aureus* isolates from healthy pig farmers, human controls, and pigs. Emerg Infect Dis 2005;11(5):711–4.

29. van Duijkeren E, Wolfhagen MJ, Box AT, et al. Human-to-dog transmission of methicillin-resistant *Staphylococcus aureus*. Emerg Infect Dis 2004;10(12):2235–7.

30. Manian F. Asymptomatic nasal carriage of mupirocin-resistant, methicillin-resistant *Staphylococcus aureus* (MRSA) in a pet dog associated with MRSA infection in household contacts. Clin Infect Dis 2003;36(2):e26–8.

31. Sing A, Tuschak C, Hormansdorfer S, et al. Methicillin-resistant *Staphylococcus aureus* in a family and its pet cat. N Engl J Med 2008;358(11):1200–1.

32. Bender JB, Minicucci L. Diseases pets and people share. Minn Med 2007;43–7.

33. Bender J, Coughlan K, Waters K, et al. Methicillin-resistant *Staphylococcus aureus* (MRSA) infections among pets in Minnesota [abstract]. Presented program and abstracts of the 2008 international conference on emerging infectious diseases. Atlanta. Georgia. March 16–19 2008. Washington D.C.: American Society of Microbiology 2008. p. 87.

34. Jones RD, Kania SA, Rohrbach BW, et al. Prevalence of oxacillin- and multidrug-resistant Staphylococci in clinical samples from dogs: 1,772 samples (2001–2005). J Am Vet Med Assoc 2007;230(2):221–7.

35. May ER, Hnilica KA, Frank LA, et al. Isolation of *Staphylococcus schleiferi* from healthy dogs and dogs with otitis, pyoderma, or both. J Am Vet Med Assoc 2005;227(6):928–31.

36. Burke JP, Riley DK. Nosocomial urinary tract infections. In: Mayhall CG, editor. Hospital epidemiology and infection control. Baltimore: Williams & Wilkins; 1996. p. 139–53.

37. National Association of State Public Health Veterinarians 2008. Compendium of veterinary standard precautions: zoonotic disease prevention in veterinary personnel.

Available at: http://www.nasphv.org/Documents/VeterinaryPrecautions.pdf. Accessed December 10, 2008.

38. Johnson JA. Nosocomial infections. Vet Clin North Am Small Anim Pract 2002; 32(5):1101–26.

39. Kruth SA, Prescott JF, Welch MK, et al. Nosocomial diarrhea associated with enterotoxigenic *Clostridium perfringens* infection in dogs. J Am Vet Med Assoc 1989;195:331–4.

40. Wise LA, Jones RL, Reif JS, et al. Nosocomial canine urinary tract infections in a veterinary teaching hospital (1983 to 1988). J Am Anim Hosp Assoc 1990; 26(2):148–52.

41. Fox JG, Beaucage CM, Folta CA, et al. Nosocomial transmission of *Serratia marcescens* in a veterinary hospital due to contamination by benzalkonium chloride. J Clin Microbiol 1981;14:157–60.

42. Ketaren K, Brown J, Shotts EB, et al. Canine salmonellosis in a small animal hospital. J Am Vet Med Assoc 1981;179:1017–8.

43. Uhaa IJ, Hird DW, Hirsch DC, et al. Case-control study of risk factors associated with nosocomial *Salmonella krefeld* infection in dogs. Am J Vet Res 1988;49: 1501–5.

44. Weese JS, Armstrong J. Outbreak of *Clostridium difficile*–associated disease in a small animal veterinary teaching hospital. J Vet Intern Med 2003;17(6):813–6.

45. Sanchez S, McCrackin Stevenson MA, Hudson CR, et al. Characterization of multidrug-resistant Escherichia coli isolates associated with nosocomial infections in dogs. J Clin Microbiol 2002;40(10):3586–95.

46. Murtaugh RJ, Mason GD. Antibiotic pressure and nosocomial disease. Vet Clin North Am Small Anim Pract 1989;19(6):1259–74.

47. Lippert AC, Fulton RB, Parr AM, et al. Nosocomial infection surveillance in a small animal intensive care unit. J Am Anim Hosp Assoc 1988;24:627–36.

48. Johnson JA, Murtaugh RJ. Preventing and treating nosocomial infection. Part II. Wound, blood, and gastrointestinal infections. Compendium on Continuing Education for the Practicing Veterinarian 1997;19(6):693–703, 719.

49. Peterson KD, Novo R, Larweck MA, et al. Implementation of a surgical infection surveillance program at a small animal veterinary medical center (VMC). Am J Infect Control 2007;35(5):E195–6.

50. American Veterinary Medical Association. AVMA policy—judicious therapeutic use of antimicrobials. Available at: http://www.avma.org/issues/policy/jtua.asp. Accessed May, 2008.

51. American Veterinary Medical Association. AVMA policy—American Association of Feline Practitioners American Animal Hospital Association basic guidelines of judicious therapeutic use of antimicrobials. Available at: http://www.avma.org/issues/policy/jtua_aafp_aaha.asp. Accessed May, 2008.

52. American Academy of Pediatrics Subcommittee on Management of Acute Otitis Media. Diagnosis and management of acute otitis media. Pediatrics 2004;113(5): 1451–65.

53. American Academy of Pediatrics Subcommittee on Management of Sinusitis and Committee on Quality Improvement. Clinical practice guideline: management of sinusitis. Pediatrics 2001;108(3):798–808.

54. King CK, Glass R, Bresee JS, et al. Managing acute gastroenteritis among children: oral rehydration, maintenance, and nutritional therapy. MMWR Recomm Rep 2003;52(RR-16):1–16.

55. Gross P, Patel B. Reducing antibiotic overuse: a call for a national performance measure for not treating asymptomatic bacteriuria. Clin Infect Dis 2007;45(10):1335–7.

56. Perz JF, Craig AS, Coffey CS, et al. Changes in antibiotic prescribing for children after a community-wide campaign. JAMA 2002;287(23):3103–9.
57. Samore MH, Bateman K, Alder SC, et al. Clinical decision support and appropriateness of antimicrobial prescribing: a randomized trial. JAMA 2005;294(18): 2305–14.
58. Weese JS. Investigation of antimicrobial use and the impact of antimicrobial use guidelines in a small animal veterinary teaching hospital: 1995–2004. J Am Vet Med Assoc 2006;228(4):553–8.
59. DeVincent SJ, Reid-Smith R. Stakeholder position paper: companion animal veterinarian. Prev Vet Med 2006;73(2–3):181–9.
60. Secchi S, Babcock BA. Pearls before swine? Potential trade-offs between the human and animal use of antibiotics. American Agricultural Economics Association Annual Meeting, Long Beach, California, July 2002. Am J Agric Econ 2002;84(5):1279–86.
61. Cook M, Molto E, Anderson C, et al. Fluorochrome labelling in roman period skeletons from Dakhleh Oasis, Egypt. Am J Phys Anthropol 1989;80(2): 137–43.

The Human–Companion Animal Bond: How Humans Benefit

Erika Friedmann, PhD*, Heesook Son, MPH, RN

KEYWORDS

- Animal assisted therapy • Pet therapy
- Animal-assisted activities • Stress reduction • Pets
- Assistance animals • Assistance dogs • Companion animals

The human–animal bond is extremely important to most clients of small animal veterinary practices.[1] Most small animal veterinarians recognize the importance of the bond but may not have had formal training in how to incorporate this recognition into their practices. Evaluation of the bond between the pet and the owner by the veterinarian and the staff during each visit is an important step.[1] Discussing the bond and behavior issues with clients also can identify problems before they become insurmountable. Local resources for addressing bond problems can be provided to clients and posted in the office. When bonding issues are discussed and noted in the record, they can be monitored at subsequent visits. This article provides the research data regarding the human health benefits of companion animals, animal-assisted therapy, animal-assisted activities, and assistance animals; reviews measures that can be taken to enable safe pet ownership for immunocompromised individuals; and discusses the veterinarian's role in supporting immune-compromised clients and clients who have assistance animals.

Pet ownership, or just being in the presence of a companion animal, can have a positive effect on individuals' mental and physiologic health status. Most research addressing health benefits of pet ownership or companion animals focuses on reductions in distress and anxiety, decreases in loneliness and depression, and increases in exercise.[2]

The biopsychosocial model of health provides a theoretic model for understanding the interrelationship of the social, psychologic, and biologic realms of health status. Health is conceptualized as ranging from minimum to maximum in a continuous dynamic process that requires ongoing adaptation to challenges. This model emphasizes the interactive nature of the three realms. Disruptions or enhancements in any realm affect the others, and together these realms comprise health status.[3]

University of Maryland School of Nursing, 655 W. Lombard Street, Baltimore, MD 21201, USA
* Corresponding author.
E-mail address: efrie002@son.umaryland.edu (E. Friedmann).

Vet Clin Small Anim 39 (2009) 293–326
doi:10.1016/j.cvsm.2008.10.015
0195-5616/08/$ – see front matter © 2009 Elsevier Inc. All rights reserved.

The physiologic changes that accompany psychologic distress and social isolation diminish a person's health status and enhance the development and progression of chronic diseases such as heart disease and diabetes, increasing morbidity and mortality.[4,5] For example, the physiologic changes that result from depression, anxiety, and social isolation or loneliness include hyperactivity of the sympatho-adrenal-medulla system and the hypothalamic-pituitary-adrenal axis and abnormal platelet reactivity. Sympatho-adrenal-medulla hyperactivity causes increased catecholamine release, reduced heart rate variability, increased sympathetic tone, decreased myocardial perfusion, and ventricular instability. Activation of the hypothalamic-pituitary-adrenal axis causes corticosteroid release into the blood and disruption of the immune system function, enhancing vulnerability to infection and cancer.[3,5] Over the short term, these mechanisms influence responses to stressful situations or environments; over the long term they influence the development and progression of chronic diseases. Positive health outcomes associated with companion animals result from enhancement of psychosocial status and from reduction of psychosocial distress and stress responses.

Pets and companion animals seem to reduce psychosocial distress by altering the owner's perceptions and making situations and people seem more benign. Scenes containing animals are perceived as more friendly, relaxed, cooperative, constructive, safe, and humorous. People in scenes with animals also are perceived as less tense, dangerous, and threatening and as friendlier, happier, healthier, wiser, and richer than people in the same scenes without the animals.[6–8] Companion animals also improve impressions of a potentially stressful environment such as a workplace[8] or a hospital.[9] In contrast, animals culturally associated with fear elicited negative feelings and stress responses.[10]

EFFECT OF ANIMALS ON SOCIAL INTERACTION AND HEALTH

Animal companions facilitate human companionship and decrease loneliness and social isolation (**Table 1**). Dogs act as social lubricants by encouraging strangers to meet and talk[11,12] and providing a neutral topic of conversation for new acquaintances.[13] Pets alleviate loneliness across the human spectrum from homeless children[14] to single women living alone[15] and community-living adults.[12]

The impact of pet ownership on health seems to be most important for highly stressed or socially isolated individuals.[15–17] Among patients who have HIV/AIDS, but not the entire gay-bisexual community, pet owners were less depressed than nonowners.[17] Socially isolated women were lonelier without a pet than with a pet; loneliness did not differ according to pet ownership for married women.[15] Dog ownership moderated the impact of psychologic distress on the frequency of physician contacts, even after accounting for the effects of health status, depressed mood, and demographic factors.[16]

Studies suggesting that pet ownership is associated with health benefits must be interpreted cautiously, because they show associations but not causal relationships (**Table 2**). Differences in outcomes could be related to determinants of pet ownership rather than the effects of the pets. Pet ownership was related to proxies for health status including medical visits, number of health problems, and functional status. Health insurance records of older Americans[16] demonstrated that pet owners made fewer medical visits than nonowners; however, there was no significant difference in the use of health care providers between Australian pet owners and nonowners.[18–20] In a longitudinal study, which provides stronger evidence of causality, Australian and German pet owners made about 15% fewer medical visits than nonowners.[21]

Table 1
Studies of the effects of pets on social interactions published from 1990 to the present

First Author	Participants	Design	Animal-Related Situation	Outcomes	Results
McNicholas[11]	One participant-observer	Ethologic observation	Researcher accompanied by dog during her daily routines	Social interactions	Frequency of social interactions, especially interactions with strangers, was higher when the researcher was accompanied by a dog.
Wood[12]	Random survey of 399 participants; 200 were pet owners	Telephone survey	Not applicable	Social interactions and sense of community	Pet owners were less likely to be lonely, found it easier to get to know people, and were more likely to be civically engaged than pet non-owners.
Rogers[13]	12 elderly persons; 6 were dog owners	Quasi-experimental; repeated measures and qualitative analysis	The dog owners walked with the dog	Focal point of conversation	Dogs were a primary focus of conversation. Dog owners reported less dissatisfaction with their social, physical, and emotional states.
Rew[14]	32 homeless youths	Qualitative study	Not applicable	Strategies for coping with loneliness	Most participants (81%) identified dogs as companions that provided unconditional love, reduced loneliness, and improved their health status.
Zasloff[15]	148 adult female students; 59 were pet owners	Cross-sectional survey	Not applicable	Loneliness scores	No differences between pet owners and pet non-owners. Women living alone were more lonely than those living with pets only, with other people and with pets, and with other people but not with pets.

Table 2
Summary of nonexperimental studies of pet ownership and health outcomes published from 1990 to the present

First Author	Participants	Design	Outcomes	Results
Jorm[18]	Random sample of 594 Australian adults, age ≥ 70 years; 169 were pet owners	Cross-sectional survey	Health service use, blood pressure, cognitive status	There were no differences between pet owners and pet non-owners on the physical or mental health measures or in Medicare visits to general practitioners or specialists.
Parslow[19]	Random sample of 5079 Australian adults aged 40–44 and 60–64 years; 2892 were pet owners	Cross-sectional survey	Risk factors for heart disease, health status	Pet owners had higher diastolic blood pressure than pet non-owners; there were no differences in systolic blood pressure. Pet owners also had higher body mass index, were more likely to smoke, and undertook milder physical activity compared than pet non-owners.
Parslow[20]	Random sample of 2551 Australian adults aged 60–64 years; 1240 were pet owners	Cross-sectional survey	Quality of life, personality, medication use, health service use	Pet owners had poorer physical and mental quality of life scores and higher rates of use of pain relief medication compared with pet non-owners. There was no relationship between pet ownership and number of general practitioner visits.
Headey 2007[21]	Data from national surveys in Germany (n = 9723) and Australia (n = 1246)	Longitudinal surveys	Health service use	Pet owners made about 15% fewer annual doctor visits than pet non-owners, even after controlling for gender, age, marital status, income, and other variables related to heath.
Anderson[23]	5641 attendees at a screening clinic; 784 were pet owners	Cross-sectional survey	Heart disease risk factors and physical exercise behavior	Men: pet owners had lower plasma cholesterol, triglycerides, and systolic blood pressure than pet non-owners. Women >40 years old: pet owners had lower systolic blood pressure than pet non-owners. Dog owners exercised more than owners of other pets and pet non-owners.

Study	Subjects	Study design	Measure	Results
Bauman[25]	894 adults in New South Wales, Australia	Cross-sectional survey	Dog walking hours per week	Dog owners walked 18 minutes per week more than dog non-owners. More than half of the dog owners did not walk their dogs and were less likely than dog non-owners to meet recommended physical activity levels for health benefits.
Dembicki[22]	127 senior citizens attending a meal program; 44 were pet owners	Cross-sectional survey	Heart disease risk factors and physical exercise behavior	Pet owners had lower serum triglyceride levels than pet non-owners Dog owners walked more than dog non-owners.
Siegel[16]	938 Medicare enrollees in a health maintenance organization; 345 were pet owners	Cross-sectional study	Medical contacts	Pet owners had fewer medical visits and patient-initiated medical contacts than pet non-owners. Psychosocial distress was correlated with number of medical contacts among pet non-owners but not among pet owners.
Friedmann[27]	92 patients in a coronary care unit; 53 were pet owners	Longitudinal cohort	Survival rates	Greater 1-year survival rate for pet-owners than for pet non-owners. Pet ownership was an independent predictor of survival after controlling for disease severity and social support.
Siegel[17]	708 HIV-positive homosexual and bisexual men; 361 were pet owners	Cross-sectional survey	Depression	Pet owners were less depressed than pet non-owners.
Friedmann[28]	369 patients who had ventricular arrhythmias after myocardial infarction; 103 were pet owners	Longitudinal cohort	Survival	Pet ownership and social support were independent predictors of 1-year survival after controlling for disease severity. Dog ownership was a predictor of survival after controlling for disease severity and social support.
Rajack[29]	454 patients admitted to a hospital for a myocardial infarction; 163 were pet owners	Longitudinal observational	6-month survival, hospital readmission	Pet ownership did not predict survival. Cat owners were more likely than pet non-owners to be readmitted for further cardiac problems or angina.
Raina[30]	1054 adults ≥ 65 years old; 286 were pet owners	Longitudinal survey	Deterioration in daily activities	Pet owners had smaller decreases in daily living activities than pet non-owners.

One classic earlier article is included because of its importance.

Differences in pet ownership patterns or culture may be responsible for the apparent discrepancies in the results of these surveys.[18–20,22,23] Pet ownership was more common among participants in some of the populations than in others, and the pet species was not always reported.

An important question is whether pet ownership causes better health or better health encourages pet ownership. A landmark study directly demonstrated the positive impact of obtaining a pet on a person's health by comparing the physical and mental health status of people who adopted pets from a shelter and a control group over a 6-month period.[24] Compared with the control group, adopters experienced significantly fewer minor health problems including headaches, hay fever, and painful joints, and decreases in mental health problems associated with ill health after adopting the pets (**Fig. 1**).

Pet ownership may protect people from developing coronary heart disease or slow its progression. Pet owners had lower levels of cardiovascular risk factors such as serum triglyceride and blood pressure than nonowners in two population surveys[22,23] but not in two others.[18–20] Dog owners exercised more than other study participants.[22,23,25] Furthermore, the walking that people do with their dogs may be more stimulating to the cardiovascular system, as indicated by a higher heart rate variability, than walking alone.[26]

Many longitudinal studies have demonstrated the association of pet ownership with cardiovascular health and functional status (**Table 2**). In a groundbreaking study, pet ownership was associated positively with 1-year survival of patients admitted to a coronary care unit (**Fig. 2**).[27] In a larger study, pet ownership, and dog ownership in particular, was associated with increased 1-year survival rates in patients hospitalized for coronary heart disease, even after accounting for disease severity and social support.[28] Dog owners were approximately 7.6 times more likely than those who did not own a dog to be alive at 1 year; cat ownership was not related to survival.[28] Cat owners were more likely than people who did not own pets to be readmitted within 6 months for further cardiac problems or angina, suggesting that cat ownership might have a different health impact than dog ownership.[29] The difference between dog and cat owners is inconclusive; it may be caused by confounding factors[28] or be a spurious statistical association.[29] In a separate longitudinal study, older adults' ability to complete activities of daily living decreased less in 1 year among dog and cat owners than among nonowners.[30]

Dog and cat ownership might have different associations with health status, as evidenced by cross-sectional[22,23,25,31] and longitudinal studies.[16,24,28,29] For example, cats, but not dogs, provided significant social support to their HIV-positive owners.[31] The mechanisms for differences in health status of dog and cat owners, as well as which aspects of health might be affected differentially by these animals, remain to be evaluated. One contributor to enhanced health, exercise, does differ with the pet type. Acquiring a dog led to significant increases in exercise compared with acquiring a cat or not acquiring a pet (**Fig. 3**).[24] As noted previously, several surveys indicate that dog owners exercise more than owners of other pets or pet nonowners.[22,23,25]

It is possible that pet species differ in their contributions to their respective owners' health, and this possibility raises questions about individual differences that may influence a person's choice of a pet. Lifestyles may influence an individual's choice of a pet, rather than result from acquiring a particular type of pet.[24] Differences between dog and cat owners generally were limited to the amount of exercise the individuals engage in.[22,23] There are insufficient data from owners of other species to explore differences in the effects of these pets on human health.

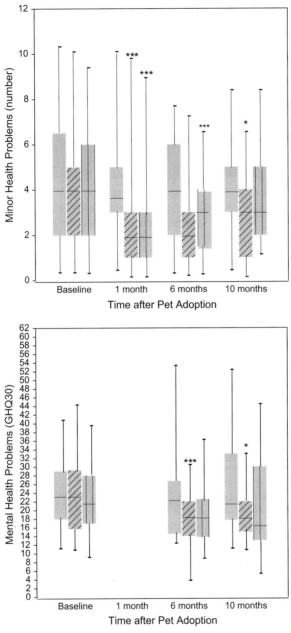

Fig. 1. Changes in reported incidence of minor health problems (*upper graph*) and mental health problems as measured with the General Health Questionnaire 30 (*lower graph*) showing median and upper and lower quartiles and minimum and maximum scores at the time of pet adoption (baseline) and 1, 6, and 10 months after pet adoption. (Significant reductions from baseline values are indicated as ***, $P < .0001$ and *, $P < .05$.) Solid color indicates the comparison group, hatched lines indicate dog adopters, and vertical lines indicate cat adopters. (*Data from* Serpell JA. Beneficial effects of pet ownership on some aspects of human health and behavior. J R Soc Med 1991;84:719.)

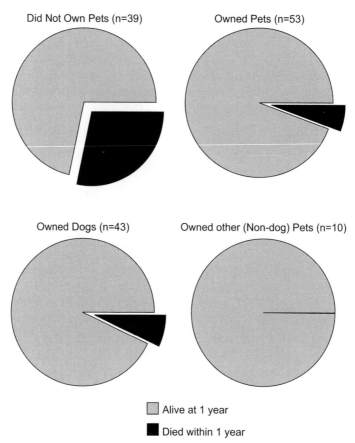

Did Not Own Pets (n=39)   Owned Pets (n=53)

Owned Dogs (n=43)   Owned other (Non-dog) Pets (n=10)

Alive at 1 year
Died within 1 year

Fig. 2. One-year mortality of patients admitted to a coronary care unit according to pet ownership status at admission. Mortality was significantly lower in pet owners ($P < .01$), dog owners ($P < .05$), and dog non-owners. ($P < .05$) than in pet non-owners. (*Data from* Friedmann E, Katcher AH, Lynch JJ, et al. Animal companions and one-year survival of patients after discharge from a coronary care unit. Public Health Rep 1980;95:307–12.)

Experimental Studies of Companion Animals' Effect on Stress

Experimental studies, which provide the strongest evidence of causality, have been used to demonstrate the effects of the presence of and interaction with companion animals on stress indicators and on stress responses (**Table 3**). Many of these studies compared people's physiologic responses or behaviors when a pet or friendly animal, usually a dog, was or was not present. These studies examined differences over the short term during specific tasks. Only studies published from 1990 to the present are included here; earlier studies are reviewed elsewhere.[2]

Looking at or observing familiar animals or a pet was associated with decreased stress indicators for people who were familiar with the animals. The blood pressure and heart rate of chimpanzee caretakers and a snake owner were lower when watching chimpanzees[32] or a pet snake, respectively, than during periods of relaxation without the animal present.[33] In contrast, heart rate and muscle tension tended to decrease and skin temperature tended to increase among older people watching a videotape of tropical fish swimming in an aquarium compared with watching live

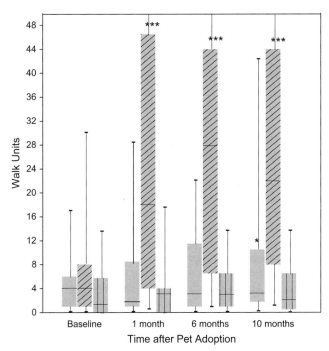

Fig. 3. Changes in reported walking units showing median and upper and lower quartiles and minimum and maximum scores at the time of pet adoption (baseline) and 1, 6, and 10 months after pet adoption. (Significant reductions from baseline values are indicated as ***, $P < .0001$ and *, $P < .05$). Solid color indicates the comparison group, hatched lines indicate dog adopters, and vertical lines indicate cat adopters. (*Data from* Serpell JA. Beneficial effects of pet ownership on some aspects of human health and behavior. J R Soc Med 1991;84:719.)

fish swimming in an aquarium or a placebo videotape. Study participants reported each stimulus as very relaxing.[34]

Touching or interacting with animals did not influence cardiac response uniformly, even with familiar animals. The blood pressure of people who did not own snakes and were not fearful of them did not differ while touching a snake and when relaxing or looking at the snake;[35] the blood pressure of a snake owner was lower when touching the snake than when watching it or during a relaxation period without the animal.[33] Despite their fondness for and lack of fear of the chimpanzees, the blood pressures and heart rates of the chimpanzees' caretakers were higher when touching or tickling the chimps through a barrier than when watching them or relaxing without the animals present.[32]

The presence of a friendly animal can moderate stress responses. Because cardiovascular stress responses vary considerably from person to person, repeated measures studies, which permit comparison of a person's response to multiple conditions, provide the best estimates of the effect of the presence of a pet or any other intervention.[2] Numerous studies indicate that it is not necessary to own a pet to obtain stress-moderating benefits from the presence of a friendly animal. The studies comparing the responses of the same individuals in the presence of friendly animals, pets, and no animals support the benefits of an animal's presence for reducing stress

Table 3
Studies of the impact of companion animals on stress indicators and stress responses published from 1990 to the present

Author	Participants	Design	Animal-Related Situation	Outcomes	Results
Motooka[26]	13 healthy volunteers	Experimental crossover design	Walking for 30 minutes with and without study dog; a subset was monitored at home, including periods of free interaction with the dog	High-frequency power values of heart rate variability	Heart rate variability increased during dog walking and was more pronounced during succeeding dog walks. At home, heart rate variability was 1.87 times greater when the dog was present and was 1.57 times greater than when walking the dog.
Eddy[32]	One chimpanzee caretaker and eight assistants	Experimental design	Touching and watching chimpanzees	Blood pressure, heart rate	Blood pressure and heart rates of a caretaker and research assistants were lower while watching the animals than during a relaxation period without the animal present.
Eddy[33]	One snake owner	Case study	Touching and watching a snake	Blood pressure	Blood pressure of the owner was lower during the snake-touching period than during the relaxation and snake-viewing periods that preceded it.
DeSchriver[34]	27 residents of a publicly subsidized housing unit	Experimental three-group pre- and posttest design	Watching a fish aquarium or a fish videotape or a placebo videotape	Heart rate, skin temperature, and muscle tension	There was a greater decrease in heart rate and muscle tension and an increase in skin temperature in the group watching the aquarium videotape than in the other groups. Participants in each group reported that the experience was relaxing.
Alonso[35]	Five persons who did not fear snakes	One group repeated measures	Holding the snake, watching the snake, or relaxing	Blood pressure, heart rate	Blood pressure and heart rates did not differ when holding snake, watching snake, or relaxing.

Study	Sample	Design	Intervention	Measures	Results
Friedmann[36]	11 community-living older adults	Experimental two-group crossover	Resting with dog present or absent and talking about daily activities	Blood pressure	Blood pressure during social stressor was 7 mmHg/2 mmHg lower when the dog was present than when the dog was absent.
DeMello[37]	50 normotensive adults	Experimental three-condition design, repeated measures	Cognitive tasks with friendly dog or goat absent, present with visual interaction, or present with tactual interaction	Blood pressure, heart rate	There was greater decrease in blood pressure and heart rate after the cognitive stressor if animal was present than if absent. There was greater reduction with visual versus tactual interaction.
Friedmann[38]	213 undergraduate students	Experimental two-group design, repeated measures	Dog present while resting and while reading aloud	Blood pressure, heart rate	Cardiovascular stress responses with dog present were lower for people who had a more positive attitude toward dogs than for those who had a more negative attitude.
Havener[39]	40 pediatric dental patients	Experimental design, repeated measures	Petting a dog while awaiting dental surgery	Behavioral distress and skin temperature	Petting dog was associated with higher skin temperature while waiting for surgery among distressed patients but not among those who were not distressed.
Wells[40]	100 volunteers	Experimental, repeated measures	Videotapes of animals were shown to participants	Blood pressure, heart rate	Blood pressure and heart rate were lower during a moderately stressful activity after viewing videos of birds, primates, and fish than after viewing control videos.

(continued on next page)

Table 3 (*continued*)

Author	Participants	Design	Animal-Related Situation	Outcomes	Results
Rajack[29]	30 women who owned dogs and 30 women who did not own dogs	Quasi-experimental two-group design, repeated measures	The presence of an animal	Heart rate, blood pressure	The heart rate and blood pressure of dog owners with their dogs present and of dog non-owners did not differ while running up and down stairs or reading aloud. Dog owners had a greater heart rate response to hearing the alarm clock.
Kingwell[41]	35 volunteer dog owners and 37 volunteer dog non-owners	Experimental two-group design, repeated measures	A friendly but unfamiliar dog was assigned randomly to the first or second half of the study	Heart rate, blood pressure, cardiac autonomic function	The presence of the dog did not influence blood pressure or heart rate either at rest or during mild mental stress. Cardiac autonomic profile was best for the dog owners with the dog present and without the dog present for the dog non-owners.
Allen[42]	45 women	Experimental three-group design, repeated measures	The presence of a dog, a friend, or no one	Cardiovascular stress responses (combination of blood pressure, heart rate, skin conductance)	Cardiovascular reactivity was reduced with the dog present versus another person, even when the person was chosen by the subject to provide support.
Allen[43]	240 married couples	Experimental four-group design, repeated measures	Participants were assigned randomly to be alone, with pet or friend (for pet non-owners), with spouse, or with spouse and pet or friend. Participants completed mental arithmetic and cold pressor tests.	Blood pressure, heart rate	Pet owners had lower resting blood pressure and smaller blood pressure increases during cold pressor tests and mental arithmetic than pet non-owners. Among pet owners, the responses to the stressful tasks were smallest when the pet was present.

Straatman[44]	36 male students 18–30 years old	Experimental two-group design, repeated measures	A friendly but unfamiliar dog sat on participants' laps during preparation and delivery of a videotaped and locally televised speech	Blood pressure, heart rate, state of anxiety	Anxiety, blood pressure, and heart rate of those with the dog on their lap and the control group members did not differ during the preparation and the speech periods, even after controlling for the effects of daily stress.
Allen[45]	48 hypertensive patients in high-stress occupations	Experimental pre- and posttest design, repeated measures	One group was assigned to get a pet, the other was not. All participants received angiotensin-converting enzyme inhibitors.	Blood pressure, heart rate, and plasma rennin activity	The groups' cardiovascular responses to mental stress did not differ before intervention; 6 months later, the stress responses were lower in those who received pets than in those who did not. In both groups, resting blood pressure was lower 6 months after the interventio but did not differ between groups.

responses.[2] In a group of 11 community-living older adults who had mild hypertension, blood pressures while talking about their daily lives were 7 mmHg/2 mmHg lower with a companion animal present than without a companion animal present.[36] The blood pressures and heart rates of normotensive adults decreased more after a cognitive stressor if a friendly goat or dog was present than if it was not present.[37] Individuals' stress responses to the presence of animals varied according to attitudes toward animals and the situation. Cardiovascular stress responses with a dog present were significantly lower for people with a more positive attitude toward dogs than for those with a less positive attitude.[38] Among pediatric patients waiting for dental surgery, petting a dog was associated with lower physiologic arousal, as assessed by finger skin temperature, for children who indicated distress but not for children who were not distressed.[39] An elegant study, in which blood pressure and heart rate were lower during a moderately stressful activity after viewing videos of birds, primates, or fish than after control conditions, demonstrated the potential for many species to reduce stress responses.[40]

Evidence for moderation of the stress response by the presence of a friendly companion animal is less consistent when comparing different individuals' responses to the animal's presence. Blood pressure and heart rate responses to a number of everyday mild stressors did not differ between dog owners with their dogs present and nonowners.[29,41] The cardiovascular stress response to a standard laboratory stress task, however, was lower for subjects who had a friendly but unfamiliar dog present than for those who had another person present, even when the person was chosen by the subject to provide support.[42] Extending this study, the cardiovascular stress responses of married pet owners were smaller when only their pet was present than in several other conditions, including the presence of the spouse.[43]

In some instances, interaction with an animal may interfere with task completion and even increase stress rather than moderating it. Placing an unfamiliar small dog in the laps of men preparing for and presenting a 4-minute videotaped and locally televised speech did not lead to lower cardiovascular stress responses than in men without a dog in their lap.[44] The reduction in blood pressure after a cognitive task was greater when the person observed an unfamiliar dog or goat than when the person interacted with the animal.[37]

In a small clinical trial, adding a pet to a nonowner's life improved the new owner's health status. Men in a high-stress occupation who had hypertension and who were willing to keep pets were assigned randomly to obtain dogs or cats (therapy group) or not (control/usual care group). All patients received an angiotensin-converting enzyme inhibitor for hypertension. Resting blood pressures of all participants were lower after 6 months. Although the cardiovascular responses to mental stress did not differ in the groups before intervention, 6 months later the stress responses were lower in pet owners than in nonowners (**Fig. 4**).[45] This study provides the strongest evidence for direct health benefits from acquiring a pet among people who were willing to do so.

THERAPY ANIMALS

People who do not own pets or are temporarily in living situations that preclude them from having pets can still benefit from visits with therapy animals (**Table 4**). Therapy animals usually are personal pets that accompany their owners to provide supervised, goal-directed interventions to clients in hospitals, nursing homes, schools, and other therapeutic sites. Several terms are used to describe these activities including "animal-assisted activities," "animal-assisted therapy," "pet therapy," and "pet

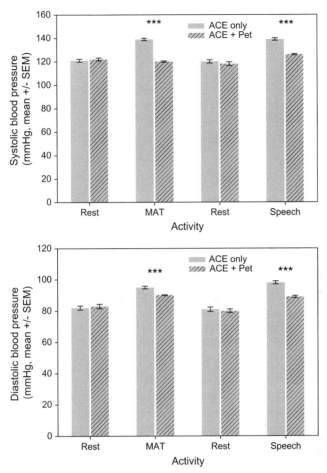

Fig. 4. Systolic and diastolic blood pressure at rest and while performing two stressful tasks, performing mental arithmetic (MAT) and speaking: (Speech), 6 months after the initiation of the angiotensin-converting enzyme inhibitor (ACE) therapy in 48 hypertensive adults; half of whom were assigned randomly to obtain pet dogs or cats in addition to taking ACE inhibitors. ***, $P < .001$. (*Data from* Allen K, Shykoff BE, Izzo JL. Pet ownership, but not ACE inhibitor therapy, blunts home blood pressure responses to mental stress. Hypertension 2001;38:815–20.)

visitation." "Animal-assisted activities" and "animal-assisted therapy" are the preferred terms. These terms have distinct meanings, as described in the following sections.

Animal-Assisted Activities

Animal-assisted activities provide motivational, educational, recreational, and/or therapeutic opportunities to enhance quality of life for groups or individuals.[46] The goals of animal-assisted activities most frequently address enhancing the social interaction or mood of individuals in an institutional setting. The benefits of animal-assisted activities are similar to those of owning a pet: improved mood[47] and decreased physiologic distress,[46,48–50] depression,[46,47] and loneliness.[51,52] The animal-assisted activities

Table 4
Studies of the effects of therapy animals published from 1990 to the present

Author	Participants	Design	Animal-Related Situation	Outcomes	Results
Lutwack-Bloom[47]	68 residents in two long-term care settings	Experimental pre- and posttest design, repeated measures	One group received visits from volunteers with a dog. The control group was visited by a person only.	Mood changes and depression	People receiving visits from volunteers with a dog had improved moods. There were no differences in depression.
Barker[48]	20 health care professionals	Experimental design, repeated measures	Visits with a therapy dog (20- versus 5-minute visits) compared with 20 minutes of rest	Serum cortisol, epinephrine, norepinephrine, salivary cortisol and IgA, and lymphocyte count	There were reductions in serum and salivary cortisol when the dog was present. There was no difference between 5-minute and 20-minute visits.
Cole[49]	76 inpatients who had advanced heart failure	Experimental three-group design, repeated measures	Therapy dog accompanied by a visitor compared with a visitor only or no visitor	Hemodynamic measure, neurohormone levels, and state anxiety	The dog group had greater decreases in systolic pulmonary artery and pulmonary capillary wedge pressures and anxiety levels than the visitor -only group and than the no-visitor group. The dog group had greater decreases in epinephrine and norepinephrine levels than the no-visitor group.
Orlandi[50]	178 oncologic patients	Quasi-experimental pre- and posttest design	Patients chose whether to have chemotherapy in the animal-assisted activities room or in the adjoining room	Anxiety, depression, somatic symptoms, arterial blood pressure, heart rate, and arterial oxygen saturation	Depression improved only in the animal-assisted activities group. Arterial oxygen saturation improved in the animal-assisted activities group but worsened in the control group.

Study	Sample	Design	Intervention	Outcome	Findings
Souter[46]	Five studies	Meta-analysis	Animal-assisted activities and animal-assisted therapy	Depression	Both animal-assisted activities and animal-assisted therapy reduced depression.
Bouchard[51]	27 pediatric oncology patients	1-year pilot project	Animal-assisted therapy with a dog present at the child's bedside for 8 hours	Client's satisfaction	Parents reported that with animal-assisted therapy, their child gained confidence, developed a friendship with the animal, and was happier. Nurses used the children's relationship with the dogs to encourage acceptance of their therapy.
Banks[52]	38 elderly persons in long-term care facilities	Experimental study	Receiving animal-assisted therapy or a robotic dog	Loneliness	Both the animal-assisted therapy and robotic dog groups were less lonely than the control group after therapy.
Banks[54]	45 residents of three long-term care facilities	Experimental three-group design	One or three animal-assisted therapy sessions per week compared with no animal-assisted therapy.	Loneliness (Version 3 of the UCLA Loneliness Scale)	Animal-assisted therapy reduced loneliness. There was no difference between the groups receiving one and three animal-assisted therapy sessions per week.
Sobo[53]	25 children in a tertiary care children's hospital	Pre- and posttest and a descriptive pilot study	Animal-assisted therapy during the child's hospitalization along with standard pharmacologic pain management. The patient decided whether to have an animal visit and the duration of the visit.	Pain perception	Animal-assisted therapy reduced perceived pain. Animal-assisted therapy may distract children from pain-related cognition and activate comforting thoughts related to companionship or home.

(continued on next page)

Table 4 (*continued*)

Author	Participants	Design	Animal-Related Situation	Outcomes	Results
Bernstein[55]	33 nursing home patients	Quasi-experimental study	Animal-assisted therapy with shelter animals brought by volunteers to group sessions compared with session of arts and crafts and snack bingo	Frequency and rates of social behaviors including conversation types and touch	During animal-assisted therapy, residents conversed with others, including the animals, as much as or more than residents receiving non–animal-assisted therapy and were more likely to initiate and to participate longer in conversations. Touching animals during animal-assisted therapy added to resident engagement in and initiation of this behavior.
Fick[56]	36 nursing home residents	Experimental study	The presence or absence of a dog during a discussion group	The frequency and types of social interactions	There was a significant increase in verbal interactions among residents when the dog was present.
Kramer[57]	18 female nursing home residents who had dementia	Experimental three-group crossover design, repeated measures	Visitor with a dog, visitor with a robotic dog, and a visitor alone	Social behaviors	Both the dog and robotic dog stimulated resident social interaction beyond that stimulated by the visitor alone.
Richeson[58]	15 nursing home residents who had dementia	Quasi-experimental pre- and postest series design with three phases	Participants interacted with the dog, reminisced about past pets, and talked to the handler and staff	Agitated behaviors and social interactions	Agitated behaviors decreased, and social interaction increased from pretest to posttest
McCabe[59]	22 patients in the Alzheimer unit of an extended health care facility	Within-participants repeated-measures design	The therapy dog was present in common areas and residents' rooms from morning to evening, except for mealtimes.	Agitation behaviors (Nursing Home Behavior Problem Scale)	Participants on the day shift showed fewer problem behaviors than those on the evening shift.

Study	Design	Intervention	Outcome Measures	Results
LaFrance[60]	One 61-year-old male patient who had aphasia	Case study, experimental repeated measures	Therapy dog accompanied patient on walk back to the ward after an animal-assisted therapy session	Overt social-verbal and social-nonverbal communication	The presence of the dog increased participant's social-verbal and social-nonverbal behavior.
Anderson[61]	Six children who had severe emotional disorders	Qualitative study, observation	A dog in the self-contained classroom	Emotional stability and learning	The dog contributed to children's overall emotional stability, improved attitudes toward school, and facilitated learning lessons in responsibility, respect, and empathy.
Esteves[62]	Three 5-to 9-year-old children who had developmental disabilities and their teacher	Case studies with repeated measures	Presence of an obedience-trained dog	Categorized social behaviors: positive/ negative, verbal/ non-verbal, and initiations/responses	Increase in overall positive initiated behaviors toward both the teacher and the dog and overall decrease in negative initiated behaviors. Social responsiveness in the classroom improved following the sessions.
Bardill[67]	30 adolescents hospitalized in a psychiatric unit	Ethnographic approach	Spontaneous interactions with a dog that was a 24-hr/d resident of the unit	People's perceptions about a given experience	The dog served as a catalyst for interactions and often was ascribed human qualities by the participants.
Barker[63]	35 adult psychiatric patients scheduled for electroconvulsive therapy	Quasi-experimental two-group design	A 15-minute session with animal-assisted therapy or a magazine before the scheduled electroconvulsive therapy	Anxiety, fear, and depression by using visual analog scales	Animal-assisted therapy reduced fear by 37% and anxiety by 18%. Animal-assisted therapy had no demonstrated effect on depression.
Barak[64]	20 elderly schizophrenic patients	Experimental two-group design	The use of cats and dogs for animal-assisted therapy or a news reading/discussion group without animal-assisted therapy	Mobility, interpersonal contact, communication, and activities of daily living (Scale for Social Adaptive Functioning Evaluation)	Total and social functioning subscale scores on the Scale for Social Adaptive Functioning Evaluation improved in the animal-assisted therapy group but not in the control group.

(continued on next page)

Table 4 (*continued*)

Author	Participants	Design	Animal-Related Situation	Outcomes	Results
Sockalingam[65]	Atypical depression in an assault victim with subsequent head injury	Clinical case study	The patient spent several hours each day with a dog over a 3-week period	Psychiatric rehabilitation	Animal-assisted therapy was effective in the psychiatric rehabilitation of an assault victim with a concurrent mood disorder.
Prothmann[68]	100 children and adolescents who had undergone inpatient psychiatric treatment	Quasi-experimental design	Each member of the treatment group had therapy dog for 30 minutes, once a week, for 5 weeks	State of mind, including vitality, intra-emotional balance, social extroversion, and alertness (Basler Befindlichkeits-Skala)	State of mind improved in the animal-assisted therapy group but not in comparison group.
Schultz[69]	63 child victims of intrafamily violence	One group; pre- and posttest design	Equine-assisted psychotherapy; learned horse grooming and practiced over 19 sessions	General level of functioning in a health-illness continuum (Children's Global Assessment of Functioning Scale)	Improvement in level of functioning was correlated with the number of sessions given.
Bizub[70]	Five persons who had longstanding histories of psychiatric disabilities	Qualitative study	Participants in a therapeutic horseback riding program for 10 weeks	The riders' experiences	By the end of the program, the riders reported augmented sense of self-efficacy and self-esteem.
Burgon[71]	Six women who had various mental health problems	Case study	Participants received weekly equine riding therapy	The riders' experiences from the therapy	The participants showed increased confidence and self-concept. The therapy aided social stimulation and led to acquisition of transferable skills.

Study	Participants	Design	Conditions	Outcome measures	Results
Limond[72]	Eight children who had Down syndrome	Experimental, counter-balanced, repeated measures design	Two conditions per session per child for 7 minutes: real dog versus imitation dog	General social behaviors (ie, looking at and responding to the adult and initiating social behaviors)	The real dog provided a more sustained focus than the imitation dog for positive and cooperative interactions with the dog and the adult.
Martin[73]	10 children who had pervasive developmental disorders	Experimental repeated-measures design	Presence of a therapy dog, a stuffed dog, or a ball while interacting with a therapist	Behavioral and verbal dimension of prosocial and nonsocial interaction	In the presence of a therapy dog, children showed a more playful mood, were more focused, and were more aware of their social environments.
Gee[74]	14 language-impaired and typical preschool children	Experimental, repeated measures	The presence of a therapy dog or no dog	Gross motor skills tasks	Children completed the tasks faster with the dog present than with the dog absent. The dog served as an effective motivator for the children.
Tissen[75]	230 third-grade children and nine teachers	Experimental three-group design, repeated measures	Three conditions: social training without dogs, social training with dogs, and dog present without social training	Social behavior, empathy, and aggression	Students' social behavior improved in all programs. Relational aggression improved in both dog groups but worsened in the group without the dog. Victim of aggression improved in the social training with dog group only.

also led to reduced perceptions of pain in children after surgery.[53] Animal-assisted activities also affect recipient behaviors by facilitating social interaction.[54–58] Both resident[59] and visiting[58] dogs reduced agitation behavior in a nursing home Alzheimer's unit.[49] Animal-assisted activities with individuals generally were more effective than animal-assisted activities with groups for improving social interaction and mood.[2]

Animal-Assisted Therapy

Animal-assisted therapy involves using animals as an integral part of a therapeutic treatment process.[46] These interventions are effective for adults and children who have psychiatric or developmental disabilities. Animals are used as co-therapists to facilitate psychotherapy or provide specific types of therapeutic interventions such as improving motor skills[60] or behavior.[61,62] Introducing dogs into psychotherapeutic interactions with psychiatric patients was effective in decreasing patient fears[63] and enhancing socialization, activities of daily living, and quality of life of adults.[64,65] Observing how children relate to animals can enrich the understanding of their current stage of development[66] and can be used to advantage in choosing appropriate therapeutic interventions. Animal-assisted therapy has been effective as a catalyst for psychotherapeutic interaction with adolescents.[67] Animal-assisted therapy sessions separate from other therapeutic interventions were effective in improving state of mind among children and adolescent psychiatric patients.[68] Therapeutic interactions with horses that included riding and caring for the animals improved confidence and self-esteem, and these improvements transferred to other areas of abused children's[69] and psychiatric patients' lives.[70,71] Animal-assisted therapy was particularly effective as an adjunctive educational intervention for improving classroom behavior of children who had emotional or developmental disabilities.[61,62,72,73] For children who had disabilities, animal-assisted therapy also was effective as a classroom adjunct for improving motor skills of preschool children[74] and teaching empathy to school-aged children.[75]

Assistance Animals

Assistance animals are trained to perform tasks for the benefit of individuals who have a variety of disabilities[76] including hearing loss,[77–79] physical disabilities,[79–81] emotional disabilities,[82] seizures disorders,[83] and diabetes.[84] Based on their importance in the functional lives of their disabled owners, Title III of the Americans with Disabilities Act of 1990 mandates that assistance or service animals be accepted in public facilities where other animals are forbidden.[79,82]

Assistance animals increase their owners' ability to function in the able-bodied world by facilitating increased exercise and mobility (**Table 5**). In telephone interviews, 81% of 404 blind owners of guide dogs reported improved mobility after obtaining the dog.[85] Adults who had spinal cord injuries who received assistance dogs reported perceptions of increased physical fitness 6 months after obtaining the dog.[81]

In addition to providing the services for which they are trained, assistance animals improve the psychosocial health of their users by decreasing their anxiety,[77,86] depression, and loneliness[78–81] and increasing their social support[78,81,85,86] and self-esteem.[79–81] Assistance dog recipients also experienced enhanced perceptions of health,[86] independence,[77,81,85] and feelings of safety.[78,79]

Special Considerations for Care of Assistance Animals

Assistance animals require special attention from their veterinarians. Although the assistance animal improves the life of the user, this role may impinge upon the animal's welfare. Dogs with hereditary disabilities such as hip dysplasia may not be able to carry out their functions as the user's mobility increases. The animal's stress level may result in poor health, inability to meet functional expectations, and deterioration of the user–assistance animal relationship. Veterinarians and their staff must be vigilant for signs of stress or overwork in assistance animals and query the user for signs of deterioration in the user–dog relationship. Client education can be effective in reducing stress and enabling a continued working relationship.

If veterinary care requires an assistance dog to be hospitalized or removed from its normal working role, the change will have major impact on the client's function and physiological status. Because the assistance animal reduces or eliminate the user's need for both paid and unpaid assistance,[80] even temporary loss of the assistance animal's role will require changes in the client's self-care. Interim arrangements for the client's well being may require consultation with social service agencies and families and delay both the initial veterinary consultation and the initiation of recommended therapy. The veterinarian's recognition of the client's difficulty in this situation is of utmost importance, because the situation may lead to extreme client distress.

ZOONOSES

Zoonotic diseases from companion animals, such as salmonellosis, giardiasis, cryptosporidiosis, bartonellosis, campylobacteriosis, and toxoplasmosis,[87] are a potential concern for anyone who comes into contact with animals. A thorough discussion of zoonotic diseases is beyond the scope of this article. The readers can refer to **Table 6** for a concise summary of the major zoonoses and to a number of excellent review articles on this subject.[87–92] Health care and long-term care facilities often are reluctant to allow assistance or therapy animals into their facilities because of concerns about infection, injuries, allergies, and other potential risks.[82,93] Addressing these valid concerns will minimize risk to vulnerable individuals while maximizing opportunities for patients to benefit from these animals.

Zoonotic diseases are of particular concern for persons who are immunocompromised. Individuals whose immune systems are compromised because of age, pregnancy, HIV/AIDS, or immunosuppressive therapy are more susceptible to zoonotic infection and are more likely to suffer serious sequelae or death as a result of infection.[87,91,92] Most pets pose little threat of transmission of zoonoses to people, however.[87] In most cases people and animals acquire zoonotic infections from the environment simultaneously and independently, not from each other.[87] Client education is extremely effective in reducing the risk from zoonotic diseases, even for high-risk individuals such as the immunocompromised.

Normal precautionary measures, such as hand washing after contact with any pet (including fish, reptiles, birds, and small rodents) and before handling food and avoiding contact with animal feces, will prevent transmission of most zoonoses. Avoidance of cat scratches or bites can prevent transmission of bartonellosis, which is carried by about 40% of pet cats without any sign of illness.[87] A person who is immunocompromised should have someone else clean litter boxes and cages/habitats.[91,94] Scooping cat litter boxes daily and placing them away from food-preparation areas will minimize household exposure to fecal material. Lining litter boxes and birdcages with disposable liners and discarding the liners weekly also minimizes exposure to feces. Transmission of infections to high-risk individuals from fish can be prevented by wearing gloves while cleaning aquariums or handling fish. Reptiles present a significant risk of zoonotic transmission of *Salmonella* infections. If high-risk individuals must keep reptiles, wearing protective gloves when touching the animals or cleaning their cages reduces the risk of zoonoses.[94,95]

Table 5
Studies of the effects of assistance animals published from 1990 to the present

Author	Participants	Design	Animal-Related Situation	Outcomes	Results
Guest[77]	51 deaf or hard-of-hearing persons	One group, longitudinal	A hearing dog trained for a number of sounds was placed with each of the participants	Tension, depression, aggression, vigor, fatigue, confusion, and overall mood disturbance	Participants reported reductions in hearing-related problems such as improved response to environmental sounds; reduced tension, anxiety, and depression; and improved social involvement and independence.
Hart[78]	39 deaf persons with hearing dogs and 15 prospective owners	Cross-sectional survey	Participants were asked to answer the outcome variables regarding a hearing dog	Loneliness, changes in social interactions, and life stress	Owners felt safer and were less lonely after obtaining their dog. Owners also felt the dogs changed their interactions with the hearing community and neighbors; few prospective owners foresaw these effects.
Valentine[79]	24 owners of service dogs and seven trainers	Cross-sectional survey	Questionnaires and interviews about a service dog	Psychosocial benefits and liabilities of service dog ownership	Respondents reported feeling less lonely, less depressed, more capable, safer, more assertive, more content, more independent, and having increased self-esteem.
Allen[80]	48 persons who had severe and chronic ambulatory disability requiring wheelchairs	Randomized clinical trial	Experimental group members received trained service dogs 1 month after the study began	Physiologic, social, demographical, and economical improvement	Dog recipients had increases in self-esteem, internal locus of control, and physiologic well being within 6 months of receiving dogs. School attendance and employment increased, and the amount of assistance needed decreased.

Study	Sample	Design	Intervention	Measures	Results
Rintala[81]	22 adults who had spinal cord injuries	Qualitative and quantitative methods: one group pre- and posttest compared with a retrospective group	The placement of a service dog with individuals who had mobility impairments	Expectations, perceived benefits and negative aspects, and satisfaction with service dogs	Participants with dogs reported perceptions of increased physical fitness 6 months after obtaining dogs. Self-esteem, mobility, safety, frequency of public outings, contacts with others in public, and feeling needed and independent also increased.
Strong[83]	10 patients who had epilepsy with tonic-clonic seizures	One group longitudinal	The placement of seizure-alert dogs	Seizure frequency	There was a reduction in seizure frequency 12–24 weeks after receiving a dog compared with the 12 weeks before receiving the dog. Only one patient showed no improvement.
Whitmarsh[85]	404 visually impaired owners of guide dogs and 427 visually impaired non-owners of guide dogs	Cross-sectional survey	Quantitative and qualitative questions about guide dogs	Perceptions of guide dog ownership among owners and non-owners	Guide dog owners reported increased mobility, independence, walking, security, companionship, friendliness from others, and offers of help after obtaining dog. They also reported increased responsibility, inconvenience, and unwanted attention from people.
Lane[86]	57 recipients of a dog for the disabled	Cross-sectional survey	Participants completed a questionnaire regarding their dog	Satisfaction with their dog, commitment to the dog's welfare, and other life changes	Participants reported an increased sense of social integration, enhancement to self-perceived health, and an affectionate, often supportive, relationship with their dog.

Table 6
Zoonoses potentially transmitted by pets and petting/farm animals

Disease	Animal Species	Organism	Category	Transmission	Signs and Symptoms
Arthropod infections (skin mites and ticks)	Rabbits, rodents	*Sarcoptes mange mite Cheyletidae Dermanyssidae Macronyssidae Trixacarus caviae*	Parasite	Direct contact with infected animals	Temporary dermatitis Human infestation is transitory because mites do not reproduce on human skin.
Ascaridiasis (Roundworm infection)	Dogs Cats	*Toxicara canis Toxicara catis Toxascaris leonina*	Parasite	Ingestion of infective eggs in environment	Dependent on organ damaged during larval migration: visual, neurologic, or tissue damage
Bartonellosis ("cat scratch disease")	Cats	*Bartonella henselae*	Bacteria	Cat scratch, bite	Skin lesions, infection at point of injury, lymphadenopathy
Campylobacteriosis	Cats, dogs, ferrets, farm animals, horses	*Campylobacter*	Bacteria	Generally spread by eating or drinking contaminated food or water or unpasteurized milk and by direct or indirect contact with fecal material from an infected person, animal, or pet (especially puppies and kittens)	Mild to severe infection of the gastrointestinal system, watery or bloody diarrhea, fever, abdominal cramps, nausea and vomiting; a rare complication of *Campylobacter* infection is Guillain-Barre syndrome.
Cryptococcosis	Wild birds (pigeons)	*Cryptococcus neoformans*	Mycotic	Isolated from the soil, usually in association with bird droppings Inhalation of airborne yeast cells and/or basidiospores	Initial pulmonary infection usually is asymptomatic. Most patients present with disseminated infection, especially meningoencephalitis.

Disease	Animal source	Agent	Type	Transmission	Signs/Symptoms
Cryptosporidiosis	Cats, dogs, farm animals, ferrets, horses	*Cryptosporidium*	Parasite	Fecal-oral route	Watery diarrhea, accompanied by abdominal cramps; nausea, vomiting, fever, headache, and loss of appetite also may occur. Rarely, the parasite can cause an inflammation of the gall bladder or infect the lining of the respiratory tract causing pneumonia.
Dermatophytosis (ringworm)	Cats, cows, dogs, goats, horses, pigs, rabbits, rodents	*Microsporum cani* *Trichophyton mentagrophytes*	Mycotic	Direct or indirect contact with asymptomatic animals or with skin lesions of infected animals, contaminated bedding	Often mild, self-limiting scaling, redness, and occasionally vesicles or fissures
Escherichia coli	Cows	*Escherichia coli 0157*	Bacteria	Ingestion of contaminated food, fecal-oral route	Severe, bloody diarrhea; kidney failure
Giardiasis	Dogs, ferrets	*Giardia intestinalis* (*Giardia lambia*)	Parasite	Ingestion of contaminated water or food, fecal-oral route	Diarrhea, fever, severe abdominal cramps
Hookworm	Cats, dogs	*Ancylostoma canium* *Ancylostoma brasiliense* *Ancylostoma tubaeform* *Uncinaria stenocephala*	Parasite	Ingestion of infective eggs or contact with contaminated soil	Pruritic skin lesions; intestinal bleeding; swelling and pain
Influenza	Ferret	*Influenza virus*	Viral	Via aerosol from infected ferret	Fever, muscle aches, headache
Mycobacteriosis	Fish	*Mycobacterium marinum*	Bacteria	Aquarium water: localized infections following access through broken skin	Skin lesions, disseminated disease in immunocompromised patients
Pasteurellosis	Rabbit rodents	*Pasteurella multocida*	Bacterial	Bites/scratches (bacteria found in mouth of animals)	Cutaneous infections, bacteremia

(continued on next page)

Table 6 (*continued*)

Disease	Animal Species	Organism	Category	Transmission	Signs and Symptoms
Psittacosis	Birds	*Chlamydophila psittaci* (formerly *Chlamydia psittaci*)	Bacteria	Inhalation of dried secretions from infected birds	Fever, headache, muscle aches, and a dry cough pneumonia
Rhodococcus equi	Horses	*Rhodococcus* spp	Bacteria	*R. equi* is found readily in soil, especially where domesticated livestock graze. Infection in humans derives from environmental exposure.	Pneumonia, pulmonary abscesses
Salmonellosis	Reptiles, birds, cats, chicks, dogs, ducklings, ferrets, fish, horses, rabbits	*Salmonella*	Bacteria	Ingestion of foods contaminated with animal feces. Fecal–oral route	Acute gastroenteritis with sudden onset of abdominal pain, diarrhea, nausea, and fever. May lead to septicemia.
Tapeworm	Cats, dogs, rabbits, rodents	*Dipylidium*	Parasite	Ingestion of infected flea	Proglottids are passed in feces or are found around the anus, causing itching
Toxoplasmosis	Cats	*Toxoplasma gondii*	Parasite	Ingestion of raw or undercooked infected meat, especially pork, lamb, or raw milk containing the parasite. The parasite is shed primarily in the feces of infected cats. Humans can become infected by the ingestion of food, water, or dirt contaminated with cat feces. Toxoplasmosis also can be acquired through a transplacental infection, when an infected mother passes the infection to her fetus	Flulike symptoms, lymphadenopathy

From Hemsworth S, Pizer B. Pet ownership in immunocompromised children—a review of the literature and survey of existing guidelines. Eur J Oncol Nurs 2006;10:120–2; with permission.

The potential for transmission of food-borne or environmental zoonotic agents also should be minimized. Feeding pets only high-quality commercial pet food or fully cooked and/or pasteurized food will avoid exposure to food-borne diseases. Pets must be prevented from drinking from toilets and eating out of garbage cans or unknown locations. Keeping pets in private outdoor areas prevents them from carrying feces from other animals and environments back to their human families.[91,94]

Preventing pet diseases prevents the transmission of diseases from pets to their owners.[91,94] Enhanced preventive care is essential for pets of immunocompromised clients. This care includes annual veterinary checkups, controlling fleas and ticks aggressively, keeping vaccinations current, neutering the pet, and planning for the pet's future care.[92,94] It is essential to emphasize to the client the importance of isolating themselves immediately from pets with diarrhea and of bringing a pet to the veterinarian at the first sign of any illness. Additionally, fecal diagnostic testing for *Salmonella* spp, *Campylobacter* spp, *Giardia intestinalis*, and *Cryptosporidium* spp is indicated during routine visits and whenever a pet experiences diarrhea.[91]

CLIENT EDUCATION

Physicians have begun to recognize the importance of the human–animal bond and to understand patients' reluctance to remove pets from their homes. Physicians often are not very familiar or comfortable with discussing zoonoses, but most patients do not seek information from veterinarians about their own health.[96] Veterinarians are valuable resources to physicians who treat immunocompromised individuals. Thus collaboration between veterinarians and physicians is crucial to enable clients/patients to keep their pets and obtain the benefits pets provide while minimizing any risks to their health.[91,94]

Providing pamphlets about appropriate veterinary and human health precautions to minimize zoonotic disease transmission in physician as well as veterinary waiting rooms is an appropriate collaborative effort between veterinarians and physicians. Veterinarians must provide information about zoonosis prevention to all clients as part of routine veterinary care. Clients who are at high risk might not identify themselves. Clients who are at not at high risk may expose high-risk individuals to their pets and their homes. Veterinarians also might want to post information about national and or local organizations that help immunocompromised individuals keep their pets. A list of agencies as well as other resources can be obtained from the Healthy Pets Healthy People website at http://www.lgvma.org/hphp/hphp_text.html. The Center for Disease Control and Prevention has a free brochure, "Preventing Infections from Pets," at http://www.cdc.gov/hiv/resources/brochures/print/pets.htm; it is available in Spanish at http://www.cdc.gov/hiv/spanish/resources/brochures/print/pets.htm.

SUMMARY

Research documents the positive impact of pets and animal companions on the health of their owners and of people participating in animal-assisted therapy or animal-assisted activities. In the short term, companion animals improve people's perceptions of situations and the people in them; over the longer term, pets can influence the development or progression of chronic diseases. Research demonstrates that companion animals reduce individuals' stress responses to stressful situations or environments. The support people feel from pets can be of particular value to socially isolated individuals. The veterinarian and staff play an important role in helping evaluate and maintain the health of the bond between the pet and the owner. Individuals at risk for zoonoses generally want to keep their pets and are not willing to give them up. Communication between physicians and veterinarians, appropriate handling of pets, and extra attention to the animals' veterinary care enable continued pet ownership.

REFERENCES

1. Martin F, Taunton A. Perceived importance and integration of the human-animal bond in private veterinary practice. J Am Vet Med Assoc 2006;228:522–7.
2. Friedmann E, Tsai C-C. The animal-human bond: health and wellness. In: Fine AH, editor. Handbook on animal assisted therapy: theoretical foundations and guidelines for practice. 2nd edition. San Diego (CA): Academic Press; 2006. p. 95–117.
3. Thomas SA, Chapa DW, Friedmann E, et al. Depression in patients with heart failure: prevalence, pathophysiological mechanisms, and treatment. Crit Care Nurse 2008;28:40–55.
4. McEwen BS. Stress, adaptation, and disease. Allostasis and allostatic load. Ann N Y Acad Sci 1998;840:33–44.
5. Sterling P. Principles of allostasis: optimal design, predictive regulation, pathophysiology and rational therapeutics. In: Shulkin J, editor. Allostasis, homeostasis, and the costs of adaptation. Cambridge (MA): MIT Press; 2003.
6. Friedmann E, Lockwood R. Validation and use of the animal thematic apperception test. Anthrozoos 1991;4:174–83.
7. Rossbach KA, Wilson JP. Does a dog's presence make a person appear more likeable? Anthrozoos 1992;5:40–51.
8. Schneider MS, Harley LP. How dogs influence the evaluation of psychotherapists. Anthrozoos 2006;19:128–42.
9. Caprilli S, Messeri A. Animal-assisted activity at A. Meyer Children's Hospital: a pilot study. Evid Based Complement Alternat Med 2006;3:379–83.
10. Globisch J, Hamm AO, Esteves F, et al. Fear appears fast: temporal course of startle reflex potentiation in animal fearful subjects. Psychophysiology 1999;36: 66–75.
11. McNicholas J, Collis GM. Dogs as catalysts for social interactions: robustness of the effect. Br J Psychol 2000;91(Pt 1):61–70.
12. Wood L, Giles-Corti B, Bulsara M. The pet connection: pets as a conduit for social capital? Soc Sci Med 2005;61:1159–73.
13. Rogers J, Hart LA, Boltz RP. The role of pet dogs in casual conversations of elderly adults. J Soc Psychol 1993;133:265–77.
14. Rew L. Friends and pets as companions: strategies for coping with loneliness among homeless youth. J Child Adolesc Psychiatr Nurs 2000;13:125–32.
15. Zasloff RL, Kidd AH. Loneliness and pet ownership among single women. Psychol Rep 1994;75:747–52.
16. Siegel JM. Stressful life events and use of physician services among the elderly: the moderating role of pet ownership. J Pers Soc Psychol 1990;58:1081–6.
17. Siegel JM, Angulo FJ, Detels R, et al. AIDS diagnosis and depression in the Multicenter AIDS Cohort Study: the ameliorating impact of pet ownership. AIDS Care 1999;11:157–70.
18. Jorm AF, Jacomb PA, Christensen H, et al. Impact of pet ownership on elderly Australians' use of medical services: an analysis using Medicare data. Med J Aust 1997;166:376–7.
19. Parslow RA, Jorm AF. Pet ownership and risk factors for cardiovascular disease: another look. Med J Aust 2003;179:466–8.

20. Parslow RA, Jorm AF, Christensen H, et al. Pet ownership and health in older adults: findings from a survey of 2,551 community-based Australians aged 60–64. Gerontology 2005;51:40–7.
21. Headey B, Grabka M. Pets and human health in Germany and Australia: national longitudinal results. Soc Indic Res 2007;80:297–311.
22. Dembicki D, Anderson J. Pet ownership may be a factor in improved health of the elderly. J Nutr Elder 1996;15:15–31.
23. Anderson W, Reid C, Jennings G. Pet ownership and risk factors for cardiovascular disease. Med J Aust 1992;157:298–301.
24. Serpell JA. Beneficial effects of pet ownership on some aspects of human health and behaviour. J R Soc Med 1991;84:717–20.
25. Bauman AE, Russell SJ, Furber SE, et al. The epidemiology of dog walking: an unmet need for human and canine health. Med J Aust 2001;175:632–4.
26. Motooka M, Koike H, Yokoyama T, et al. Effect of dog-walking on autonomic nervous activity in senior citizens. Med J Aust 2006;184:60–3.
27. Friedmann E, Katcher AH, Lynch JJ, et al. Animal companions and one-year survival of patients after discharge from a coronary care unit. Public Health Rep 1980;95:307–12.
28. Friedmann E, Thomas SA. Pet ownership, social support, and one-year survival after acute myocardial infarction in the Cardiac Arrhythmia Suppression Trial (CAST). Am J Cardiol 1995;76:1213–7.
29. Rajack LS. Pets and human health: the influence of pets on cardiovascular and other aspects of owners' health. Cambridge (UK): University of Cambridge; 1997.
30. Raina P, Waltner-Toews D, Bonnett B, et al. Influence of companion animals on the physical and psychological health of older people: an analysis of a one-year longitudinal study. J Am Geriatr Soc 1999;47:323–9.
31. Castelli P, Hart LA, Zasloff RL. Companion cats and the social support systems of men with AIDS. Psychol Rep 2001;89:177–87.
32. Eddy TJ. Human cardiac responses to familiar young chimpanzees. Anthrozoos 1995;4:235–43.
33. Eddy TJ. RM and Beaux: reductions in cardiac activity in response to a pet snake. J Nerv Ment Dis 1996;184:573–5.
34. DeSchriver MM, Riddick CC. Effects of watching aquariums on elders' stress. Anthrozoos 1991;4:44–8.
35. Alonso Y. Cardiovascular responses to a pet snake. J Nerv Ment Dis 1999;187:311–3.
36. Friedmann E, Thomas SA, Cook LK, et al. A friendly dog as potential moderator of cardiovascular response to speech in older hypertensives. Anthrozoos 2007;20:51–63.
37. DeMello LR. The effect of the presence of a companion-animal on physiological changes following the termination of cognitive stressors. Psychology and Health 1999;14:859–68.
38. Friedmann E, Zuck Locker B, Lockwood R. Perception of animals and cardiovascular responses during verbalization with an animal present. Anthrozoos 1990;6:115–34.
39. Havener L, Gentes L, Thaler B, et al. The effects of a companion animal on distress in children undergoing dental procedures. Issues Compr Pediatr Nurs 2001;24:137–52.
40. Wells DL. The effect of videotapes of animals on cardiovascular responses to stress. Stress and Health 2005;21:209–13.
41. Kingwell BA, Lomdahl A, Anderson WP. Presence of a pet dog and human cardiovascular responses to mild mental stress. Clin Auton Res 2001;11:313–7.

42. Allen KM, Blascovich J, Tomaka J, et al. Presence of human friends and pet dogs as moderators of autonomic responses to stress in women. J Pers Soc Psychol 1991;61:582–9.

43. Allen K, Blascovich J, Mendes W. Cardiovascular reactivity and the presence of pets, friends and spouses: the truth about cats and dogs. Psychosom Med 2002; 64:727–39.

44. Straatman I, Hanson EKS, Endenburg N, et al. The influence of a dog on male students during a stressor. Anthrozoos 1997;10:191–7.

45. Allen K, Shykoff BE, Izzo JL. Pet ownership, but not ACE inhibitor therapy, blunts home blood pressure responses to mental stress. Hypertension 2001;38:815–20.

46. Souter MA, Miller MD. Do animal-assisted activities effectively treat depression? A meta-analysis. Anthrozoos 2007;20:167–80.

47. Lutwack-Bloom P, Wijewickrama R, Smith B. Effects of pets versus people visits with nursing home residents. J Gerontol Soc Work 2005;44:137–59.

48. Barker SB, Knisely JS, McCain NL, et al. Measuring stress and immune response in healthcare professionals following interaction with a therapy dog: a pilot study. Psychol Rep 2005;96:713–29.

49. Cole KM, Gawlinski A, Steers N, et al. Animal-assisted therapy in patients hospitalized with heart failure. Am J Crit Care 2007;16:575–85.

50. Orlandi M, Trangeled K, Mambrini A, et al. Pet therapy effects on oncological day hospital patients undergoing chemotherapy treatment. Anticancer Res 2007;27: 4301–3.

51. Bouchard F, Landry M, Belles-Isles M, et al. A magical dream: a pilot project in animal-assisted therapy in pediatric oncology. Can Oncol Nurs J 2004;14:14–7.

52. Banks MR, Willoughby LM, Banks WA. Animal-assisted therapy and loneliness in nursing homes: use of robotic versus living dogs. J Am Med Dir Assoc 2008;9: 173–7.

53. Sobo EJ, Eng B, Kassity-Krich N. Canine visitation (pet) therapy: pilot data on decreases in child pain perception. J Holist Nurs 2006;24:51–7.

54. Banks MR, Banks WA. The effects of animal-assisted therapy on loneliness in an elderly population in long-term care facilities. J Gerontol A Biol Sci Med Sci 2002; 57:M428–32.

55. Bernstein PL, Friedmann E, Malsipina A. Animal-assisted therapy enhances resident social interaction and initiation in long-term care facilities. Anthrozoos 2000;13:213–24.

56. Fick KM. The influence of an animal on social interactions of nursing home residents in a group setting. Am J Occup Ther 1993;47:529–34.

57. Kramer SC, Friedmann E, Bernstein PL. Comparison of the effect of human interaction, animal assisted therapy, and AIBO assisted therapy on long-term care residents with dementia. Anthrozoos 2009;22:43–57.

58. Richeson NE. Effects of animal-assisted therapy on agitated behaviors and social interactions of older adults with dementia. Am J Alzheimers Dis Other Demen 2003;18:353–8.

59. McCabe BW, Baun MM, Speich D, et al. Resident dog in the Alzheimer's special care unit. West J Nurs Res 2002;24:684–96.

60. LaFrance C, Garcia LJ, Labreche J. The effect of a therapy dog on the communication skills of an adult with aphasia. J Commun Dis 2007;40:215–24.

61. Anderson KL, Olson MR. The value of a dog in a classroom of children with severe emotional disorders. Anthrozoos 2006;19:35–49.

62. Esteves SA, Stokes T. Social effects of a dog's presence on children with disabilities. Anthrozoos 2008;21:5–15.

63. Barker SB, Pandurangi AK, Best AM. Effects of animal-assisted therapy on patients' anxiety, fear, and depression before ECT. J ECT 2003;19:38–44.
64. Barak Y, Savorai O, Mavashev S, et al. Animal-assisted therapy for elderly schizophrenic patients. Am J Geriatr Psychiatry 2001;9:439–42.
65. Sockalingam S, Li M, Krishnadev U, et al. Use of animal-assisted therapy in the rehabilitation of an assault victim with a concurrent mood disorder. Issues Ment Health Nurs 2008;29:73–84.
66. Melson GF. Child development and the human-companion animal bond. Am Behav Sci 2003;47:31–9.
67. Bardill N, Hutchinson S. Animal-assisted therapy with hospitalized adolescents. J Child Adolesc Psychiatr Nurs 1997;10:17–24.
68. Prothmann A, Bienert M, Ettrich C. Dogs in child psychotherapy: effects on state of mind. Anthrozoos 2006;19:265–77.
69. Schultz PN, Remick-Barlow GA, Robbins L. Equine-assisted psychotherapy: a mental health promotion/intervention modality for children who have experienced intra-family violence. Health Soc Care Community 2007;15:265–71.
70. Bizub AL, Joy A, Davidson L. "It's like being in another world:" demonstrating the benefits of therapeutic horseback riding for individuals with psychiatric disability. Psychiatr Rehabil J 2003;26:377–84.
71. Burgon H. Case studies of adults receiving horse riding therapy. Anthrozoos 2003;16:263–76.
72. Limond JA, Bradshaw JWS, Cormack KFM. Behavior of children with learning disabilities interacting with a therapy dog. Anthrozoos 1997;10:84–9.
73. Martin F, Farnum J. Animal-assisted therapy for children with pervasive developmental disorders. West J Nurs Res 2002;24:657–70.
74. Gee NR, Harris SL, Johnson KL. The role of therapy dogs in speed and accuracy to complete motor skill tasks for preschool children. Anthrozoos 2007;20: 375–86.
75. Tissen I, Hergovich A, Spiel C. School-based social training with and without dogs: evaluation of their effectiveness. Anthrozoos 2007;20:365–73.
76. Sachs-Ericsson N, Hansen N, Fitzgerald S. Benefits of assistance dogs: a review. Rehabil Psychol 2002;42:251–77.
77. Guest CM, Collis GM, McNicholas J. Hearing dogs: a longitudinal study of social and psychological effects on deaf and hard-of-hearing recipients. J Deaf Stud Deaf Educ 2006;11:252–61.
78. Hart LA, Zasloff RL, Benfatto AM. The socializing role of hearing dogs. Appl Anim Behav Sci 1996;47:7–15.
79. Valentine DP, Kiddoo M, LaFleur B. Psychosocial implications of service dog ownership for people who have mobility or hearing impairments. Soc Work Health Care 1993;19:109–25.
80. Allen K, Blascovich J. The value of service dogs for people with severe ambulatory disabilities. A randomized controlled trial. JAMA 1996;275:1001–6.
81. Rintala DH, Sachs-Ericsson N, Hart KA. The effects of service dogs on the lives of persons with mobility impairments: a pre-post study design. SCI Psychosocial Process 2002;15:70–82.
82. Duncan SL. APIC state-of-the-art report: the implications of service animals in health care settings. Am J Infect Control 2000;28:170–80.
83. Strong V, Brown S, Huyton M, et al. Effect of trained seizure alert dogs on frequency of tonic-clonic seizures. Seizure 2002;11:402–5.
84. Bergin B. Staying independent with canine help. Diabetes Self Manag 2005;22: 30, 32–30, 34.

85. Whitmarsh L. The benefits of guide dog ownership. Vis Impair Res 2005;7:27–42.
86. Lane DR, McNicholas J, Collis GM. Dogs for the disabled: benefits to recipients and welfare of the dog. Appl Anim Behav Sci 1998;59:49–60.
87. Hemsworth S, Pizer B. Pet ownership in immunocompromised children–a review of the literature and survey of existing guidelines. Eur J Oncol Nurs 2006;10: 117–27.
88. Beran GW. Zoonoses in practice. Vet Clin North Am Small Anim Pract 1993;23: 1085–107.
89. Robertson ID, Irwin PJ, Lymbery AJ, et al. The role of companion animals in the emergence of parasitic zoonoses. Int J Parasitol 2000;30:1369–77.
90. Morrison G. Zoonotic infections from pets. Understanding the risks and treatment. Postgrad Med 2001;110:24–30, 35.
91. Robinson RA, Pugh RN. Dogs, zoonoses and immunosuppression. J R Soc Health 2002;122:95–8.
92. Trevejo RT, Barr MC, Robinson RA. Important emerging bacterial zoonotic infections affecting the immunocompromised. Vet Res 2005;36:493–506.
93. Brodie SJ, Biley FC, Shewring M. An exploration of the potential risks associated with using pet therapy in healthcare settings. J Clin Nurs 2002;11:444–56.
94. AVMA Committee on the Human-Animal Bond. AVMA guidelines for responding to clients with special needs. J Am Vet Med Assoc 1995;206:961–76.
95. Angulo FJ, Glaser CA, Juranek JD, et al. Caring for pets of immunocompromised persons. J Am Vet Med Assoc 1994;205:11–8.
96. Grant S, Olsen CW. Preventing zoonotic diseases in immunocompromised persons: the role of physicians and veterinarians. Emerging Infect Dis 1999;5: 159–63.

The Impact of Companion Animal Problems on Society and the Role of Veterinarians

Victoria L. Voith, DVM, PhD

KEYWORDS

• Companion animals • Behavior problems • Animals • Society

Companion animals provide joy, companionship, comfort, and psychologic and physiologic benefits to people. But not always.

The benefits of animal companionship and the presence of animals always have been known and, more recently, have been chronicled and documented.[1–5] In the last half-century, however, compressed living spaces, the demands of busy life styles, and lack of knowledge about basic animal behavior and husbandry have converged to lay the groundwork for problems related to companion animals. Sometimes these problems are germane to only the owners and their families; at other times they affect visitors and neighbors and occasionally a wider swath of the community. All these population groups are in the purview of public health.

Why should the inability to deal with an animal's behavior that primarily affects only the immediate family be considered a public health concern? For one, the benefits of pet companionship are diminished or negated. Living with a pet with a serious behavior problem induces stress, which can take a toll on the general health of a person. Household members, such as children and the elderly, who do not have control over maintenance of the pet may be at risk for injuries and disease. Also, as Murray[6] stated, the behaviors that affect owners are the same ones that impinge on members of the community, the major difference being that in the latter case non-owners are the victims.

The most common behavior problems that prompt owners to seek help from professional animal behaviorists or veterinarians are similar worldwide.[7–12] Normal behaviors for a given species often become problematic because of environmental factors and the management practices of owners. The most prevalent problems are

College of Veterinary Medicine, Western University of Health Sciences, 309 East Second Street, Pomona, CA 91766-1854, USA
E-mail address: vvoith@westernu.edu

Vet Clin Small Anim 39 (2009) 327–345
doi:10.1016/j.cvsm.2008.10.014
0195-5616/08/$ – see front matter © 2009 Elsevier Inc. All rights reserved.

aggression toward people and other animals, elimination behavior problems, destructiveness, and excessive vocalization. Most of these problems could be ameliorated or managed successfully if the problem were diagnosed and treated correctly. Even more of these problems could be prevented if the owners only knew how to do so.

IMPACT OF THE PET ON THE INDIVIDUAL OWNER AND FAMILY

The most recent American Veterinary Medical Association (AVMA) survey of companion animal ownership in the United States indicated that 6 of 10 households owned a pet at during 2006.[13] Fifty-four percent of households had dogs, cats, or both. One in four households in the United Kingdom had dogs.[14]

In the 1980s, clients at the veterinary teaching hospital at the University of Pennsylvania filled out questionnaires asking if their dog or cat engaged in any behaviors the owners considered a problem. Approximately 40% of respondents said yes.[15,16] The dog owners listed the same problems that drive owners to seek help from animal behavior therapists: aggression, elimination, destructive behaviors, and vocalizations. Cat owners were concerned primarily with elimination behaviors, chewing plants, and scratching furniture. A 2007 survey of dog owners in a semi-rural community in England indicated that 5% of the dogs urinated in the house and 4% defecated in the house "sometimes" or "often." The authors commented that many of the owners did not answer this question, perhaps because of the sensitive nature of the problem, and postulated that the percentage of dogs that eliminate in the house might be higher.[14] Clearly many people keep pets despite behaviors the owners consider problems. The severity of most of these behaviors and the toll they levy on the owners' well being remain mostly unknown.

Animal behavioral therapists have firsthand knowledge of the stress and unhappiness that companion animal problems can bring to owners and families. In addition to strained and terminated personal relationships, there is an energy drain and the financial and psychologic distress of coping with a problem. The following scenarios are common:

- A single person returns home after the usual long day at work. She is greeted by her dog that she raised from puppyhood and loves dearly. What also greets her is the daily 30-minute chore of cleaning the bathroom or dog crate smeared with feces.
- A couple who have had a companion dog for many years recently had a baby. The dog has started growling at their firstborn, now a toddler. The parents have tried everything they can think of to ameliorate the problem and are struggling with the situation by keeping the dog and child separated. This situation is becoming a management nightmare, and the owners increasingly are worried about what might happen when the child becomes more ambulatory.

Owners who have cats that urinate in the home or dogs that are aggressive toward strangers often cease having visitors, either because people decline to come over or because the owners are too embarrassed to have company. Many people, fearing damage to the house, property, or dog itself, forego social engagements because they cannot leave their dogs alone in the evenings or weekends. A dog that is a member of the family becomes a liability when it is aggressive.

The economic and psychologic tolls of dealing with a problem pet are far from trivial.

When people seeking help for an animal's behavior problem were asked why they kept pets with serious behavior problems, the majority of both dog and cat owners answered with statements of attachment or humanitarian reasons, such as, "I love him," "She's a part of the family," "If we don't keep him, who would?' or "You wouldn't get rid of a child if s/he had a behavior problem, would you?"[17] Other times, the pet is kept because of commitment, attachment, or connection to another person. The pet may "belong" to an adult child who has left home. Sometimes the pet was shared with a deceased partner. Frequently, an elderly person may try to cope with an animal that was a surprise gift, given with the intent of providing the recipient with health benefits and companionship. A sense of obligation and a fear of offending the gift giver may compel the owner to keep the pet.

When owners who consider the pet a family member make the decision to relinquish or euthanize a problem pet, the situation resembles "Sophie's choice," requiring the sacrifice of one member of the family to benefit another. Many owners have little hope that their relinquished pets ever will be adopted.

When the field of animal behavior was relatively new, nothing was known about the type of clients who might seek the help of comparative psychologists and veterinary behaviorists,[18,19] but stereotypes existed of the "crazy people" who had pets with behavior problems. Eventually the public and veterinary medical audiences began to realize that many owners had pets with varying degrees of the same behaviors. Professionals in in the behavior field soon realized that most of their clients were sane, regardless of their income level or ability to pay. What the clients had in common was a lack of accurate knowledge regarding selecting, raising, managing, and caring for their pets. Many, however, possessed a great deal of misinformation regarding the behavior and care of their pet. Likewise the profession soon realized the stress that many of these people and their pets endured living in these situations.

There is a great need for education about animal behavior and the husbandry of companion animals. In the past few decades, there has been a swell of businesses, practices, franchises, and television programs that offer help and expertise regarding behavior problems. The quality of these resources varies widely. Almost all continuing education programs at veterinary medical conferences have presentations pertaining to the treatment, diagnosis, and sometimes prevention of behavior problems. A few land grant colleges and universities have recognized the need for accurate and useful information regarding the management of companion animals and have added courses and extension agents to help educate the public. Specialty colleges for veterinary medical animal behaviorists exist in some countries (eg, the American College of Veterinary Behaviorists in the United States).[20] Academically trained comparative psychologists, ethologists, and animal behaviorists have established a certification process for Applied Animal Behaviorists under the auspices of the Animal Behavior Society.[21]

PRACTITIONERS AND STAFF HELPING CLIENTS

Veterinarians are a respected source of information about animal matters, including behavior, and could do much to assist owners with prevention and treatment of behavior problems of their animals. Simply raising the topic of behavior with clients at some point during a routine office visit often uncovers a problem or situations that may lead to one. This opening gives the practitioner an opportunity to help the owner, either immediately or by providing the owner with other long-term options. Wellness is a concept that has been applied to routine prophylactic health visits and geriatric care. It also is a concept that can be applied to the animal's behavior.[22]

The kind of advice veterinarians and staff provide depends on their knowledge and their comfort level. Practices may concentrate on preventative measures, offering special appointments to address these topics and/or always allotting extra time during puppy and kitten visits. Some veterinarians feel confident providing assistance for specific behavior problems, such as elimination behaviors, separation anxiety, and noise phobias. Other practices have specialists on staff or work in conjunction with them. Some may limit their involvement to providing physical examinations and directing clients with animal behavior problems to other resources.

HOSPITAL POLICIES

Everyone associated with a practice should understand the practice polices regarding behavior problems and know how to field questions.[23] Specific advice should not be given over the telephone or based on brief descriptions. It is unlikely that helpful or accurate advice can be given to owners based on one or two sentences regarding a problem. It is, however, quite possible to give misinformation and detrimental advice based on brief descriptions, as illustrated by the following examples.

- A pet-owner asks the receptionist if "crating" dogs is a good way to housebreak a puppy. The receptionist answers, "Yes. Crates are a great way to housebreak dogs," adding that is how she has always housebroken her dogs. The owner buys a crate and confines the dog. She comes home to find the dog has torn its nails, and its coat is soaked with urine and feces. The problem was not a housebreaking problem.
- A client confides in a technician that his dog growls at him and asks if he should punish the dog. The technician says "By all means. Immediately, grab the dog and roll him over on his back." The client does so and is bitten.
- An owner mentions, in passing, that their cat is urinating outside the litter box. The veterinarian advises the owner to add a few more boxes to the household. When this approach fails and the client seeks advice from another veterinarian, it is discovered that the cat has glucosuria and is polydypsic and diabetic.

It may be helpful for hospital personnel to have standard phrases in their repertoire to use when queried about problems. For example:

- "There are many reasons a cat may not be using a litter box. It could be a medical problem. Would you like to make an appointment for a physical and medical work-up? Based on what we find, we can recommend options from there."
- "We don't deal with aggressive behavior problems, per se, but aggression often is linked to physical ailments. Would you like to make an appointment for a thorough physical examination? We can discuss the possibilities of behavioral consultations after that."
- "We don't offer any behavioral advice over the phone. Problems are generally more complicated that they initially appear and take some time to properly diagnose. We don't want to give you the wrong advice. A physical examination may also be warranted. Would you like to make an appointment?"

Sometimes it is beneficial for staff to role-play asking and answering typical questions. It also may be helpful to have standard statements on index cards posted near the telephones.

THE CONCEPT OF BEHAVIORAL WELLNESS IN PRACTICES

Veterinarians and their staff need to be proactive in bringing up the topic of the behavior during routine office visits, especially during puppy and kitten visits.[22,24,25] Clients may not mention problems or may be embarrassed to admit their pet is engaging in a behavior that is a problem. Some clients may think it inappropriate to bring up a behavior question during a medical appointment.[26]

Open-ended questions such as "How's your puppy's housebreaking coming along?" or "What do you do when you find your puppy has urinated or defecated in the house?" can elicit meaningful information. If the client is punishing the animal inappropriately, the clinician of course immediately should advise the client to cease that activity. Then, the clinician or staff member could say, in a nonjudgmental way, something like "That approach doesn't work well for this type of problem, and (puppies/dogs/ cats) can become defensive and aggressive when they are disciplined that way. For now, just clean up the mess." If the problem cannot be addressed at that moment, the clinician or staff member might continue, "I'm sorry. We don't have time to address this adequately right now, but would you like to make a follow-up appointment for this? In the interim, here is an article on housetraining. If things don't improve in a week, it is really important that you make an appointment, either with us or someone else, to explore this further. You also can make an appointment now if you like."

During a regular office visit, cat owners might be asked "Do mind if I ask you a few questions about your cat and his litter box? Tell me how often and exactly how you clean Fuzzy's litter box?" This provides an opening to review procedures and possibly prevent future out-of-the-box experiences. It also may reveal an existing problem that can be addressed successfully.

Making a decision about what to do with a problem, how to advise, and to whom to refer clients presupposes basic knowledge about animal behavior and companion animal behavior problems. Few veterinary schools include animal behavior in their curriculum, despite requests from the public for help from their veterinarians.[27] Self-directed learners can avail themselves of continuing education meetings and applied and clinically oriented texts,[28–32] can take animal behavior or comparative psychology courses at nearby colleges, and can study articles on behavior that appear in mainstream veterinary medical journals. Some peer-reviewed journals that focus on behavioral issues include the *Journal of Applied Animal Behavior Science*, the *Journal of Applied Animal Welfare Science*, and the *Journal of Veterinary Behavior: Clinical Applications and Research*. It is helpful, however, to have formal training in animal behavior to evaluate critically the information offered by these sources.

It is somewhat of an oxymoron that the veterinary profession encourages veterinarians to treat and diagnose behavior problems but does not require the study of animal behavior in veterinary medical curricula. One way to address this paradox would be for members of the AVMA to propose to their AVMA delegates that a requirement for animal behavior is needed in veterinary medical curricula.

REFERRING ANIMAL BEHAVIOR PROBLEMS

Practitioners may want to refer some behavior problems but have difficulty deciding to whom to refer and how to evaluate the procedures used by those offering to solve pet behavior problems. The veterinary community should be aware that the terms/titles "animal behaviorist," "applied animal behaviorist," "animal behavior consultant" or "councilor," and "dog trainer" are not licensed or legally protected terms.[33–36] Anyone can use these words to describe themselves. Although the term "animal psychologist" sometimes is used as a title or to infer expertise, the title of psychologist is a legally defined and protected descriptor. Laws and regulations regarding use of the terms "psychology," "psychologist," and related language pertaining to the field and practice of psychology are defined by state statues.[37]

There currently are only three professional animal behavior groups in the United States that require college degrees for their certified or boarded constituents.[36] The

American Registry of Professional Animal Scientists, whose members are referred to as "Diplomates," use the letters "Dpl AAB" to signify their status.[38] Diplomates must have at least a master's degree in an animal science or related field. The Animal Behavior Society certifies applied or associate applied animal behaviorists and uses the letters "CAAB" and "CAAAB" as identifiers.[21] Members must have a doctorate or Master's degree in an animal behavior field. Members of the American College of Veterinary Behaviorists are recognized by the AVMA as diplomates and use the letters "DACVB".[20] Members of this college must be veterinarians and have completed either a traditional residency or a nonconforming program in veterinary animal behavior. All these groups require additional expertise and requirements. The titles and insignias of these groups are protected and cannot be used legally by other than recognized members.

Some dog-training associations with large memberships have endorsement and certification programs. These associations are the Certification Council for Pet Dog Trainers, which was developed under the auspices of the Association of Pet Dog Trainers;[39] the National Association of Dog Obedience Instructors;[40] and the International Association of Canine Professionals.[41] The qualifications for these groups differ. Veterinarians should familiarize themselves with the requirements of each of these groups, which can be found on line.[39–41] There also are numerous other self-certifying groups of trainers or private training facilities that offer certification, graduation diplomas, and recognition of completion of their programs. When a local trainer or behavior counselor solicits referrals from practitioners, it behooves the veterinarian to determine exactly what is meant by any credentials that might be presented or alluded to.

The American Society of Veterinary Behavior is comprised of veterinarians with varying levels of expertise who share an interest in animal behavior. This association provides continuing education meetings, a list serve, newsletter, and information pertaining to animal behavior on its Web site.[42] It also provides a list of veterinarians who are interested in seeing behavior cases. This organization is a society and does not confer any type of certification or endorsement of its members.

Hetts,[33] the American Veterinary Society of Animal Behaviorists,[34] and Simpson[35] provide additional synopses of terminology and qualifications of the various categories of people who offer behavioral services. More detailed discussions about these topics have appeared in the *Journal of Veterinary Behavior: Clinical Applications and Research*.[43–46]

The type of behavior problem often dictates the type of referral. If the behavior is likely to be unrelated to any medical pathology, it may be addressed through appropriate obedience training by a capable trainer.[45] Behaviors such as not coming when called, jumping on people, pulling on the leash, and fear of a specific stimulus may fall into this category.

Certification, level of education, membership in behavior or training groups, and personal recommendations are all important when evaluating a trainer.[33,34] There is, however, no substitute for observing a trainer and watching how s/he interacts with the dog and client. It is also critical to follow up on referrals. Determining whether the trainer follows the *Guidelines for Humane Dog Training* also can be used to assess a trainer. These guidelines were developed by an interdisciplinary group of professionals in the dog training, academic, and veterinary medical fields and are available from the Delta Society.[47]

Healthy dogs with complicated behavioral problems that are in need of referral would be served best by ACVB diplomates or CAABs, if they are available. There are also, however, individual members of American Society of Veterinary Behavior and trainers who are very good at dealing with and managing severe problems successfully. The difficulty is identifying them; that responsibility is the practitioner's. Ideally, practitioners who want to refer an animal and are concerned that the problem may entail a medical component or who are uncomfortable with prescribing drug therapies should refer to or consult with an ACVB diplomate.

Regardless to whom a practitioner refers, s/he should assess the efficacy of those individuals. Obtaining follow-up information regarding the outcome of referred cases is important. One should check with the client about how the pet is doing and what techniques were used. If there is no feedback from the people to whom the pet was referred, one should call them to discuss their procedures and assess their interpersonal skills. More detailed descriptions of how to evaluate services are available.[33-36]

IMPACT OF DOMESTIC COMPANION ANIMALS ON PEOPLE OTHER THAN THE PET OWNER

In urban areas, complaints about pets and their behaviors are among the complaints most frequently voiced by members of the community.[6,48-50] Noise, excrement, damage to property, and injuries are common concerns. Other undesirable situations involving companion animals are animal hoarding, feral and roaming animals, and the overpopulation of domestic dogs and cats. All these problems affect pet owners as well as the community and rural residents as well as urban residents. The annoyances and detrimental consequences of companion animals have prompted serious proposals that would require licensing of owners to permit the privilege of owning companion animals, in addition to licensing the pets.[51,52] Obtaining an owner's license could require passing tests demonstrating knowledge about husbandry and care of pets and of regulations concerning pets.

Why do owners allow their pets to engage in disruptive and detrimental behaviors? Perhaps some are not bothered by the behaviors and/or are unaware of the effects of their pets on others. There also are cultural attitudes concerning confinement, neutering, and husbandry of domestic dogs and cats.[53,54] Some owners may empathize with or live vicariously through their pets' antics. It is possible that some owners may not care that their pets are disturbing their neighbors or actually may enjoy it. Some may look on any restrictions regarding their pets as an infringement of their individual rights and as a personal assault on themselves.

Some people seem to have little or no motivation to manage their pets.[6] It is easier to let the dog run free than to build a fence or to take the dog on walks. An added bonus is that the animal probably will urinate and defecate on someone else's property. It is easier to let the dog bark outside throughout the day than to acclimate it to the house. When there are enough complaints or the pet's behavior impinges sufficiently on the owner, the animal may be abandoned, relinquished to a shelter, or confiscated by animal control. Often there is there is no effort to retrieve the animal. It is easier to get a new one that is younger and cuter. It is a disposable society, and not all pet owners are attached to the dogs and cats that they own.

Many owners, however, simply, do not know how to prevent, manage, or change the behaviors of their animals. Some may have tried, failed, and have sunk into a state of learned helplessness.[55]

Noise Annoyance

Barking dogs rank high on the list of complaints to government officials.[48-50] Gauging by the number of magazine and on-line advertisements, barking bothers many people, owners as well as non-owners. Noise pollution and annoyance are of major concern worldwide.[56–59] The World Health Organization has identified noise as an important heath issue and lists "domestic animals such as barking dogs" as a neighborhood community or environmental noise.[59] Environmental noise is defined as "noise emitted from all sources except noise at the industrial work place".[59] Other definitions that World Health Organization uses are "Noise: sound, especially when it is unwanted, unpleasant, or loud" (Cambridge Advanced Learner's Dictionary), and "Noise pollution: environmental pollution consisting of annoying or harmful noise … called also sound pollution" (MedlinePlus Health information).[59]

Exposure to prolonged and/or intermittent barking in the community is unlikely to result in hearing loss or direct cardiovascular effects, but it can result in sleep disturbance. Sleep disturbance can have a myriad of consequences—psychophysiologic effects, decline in mental and physical performance, accidents, increased fatigue, depressed mood or sense of well being, anger, agitation, anxiety, and changes in social interactions. The uncontrollability of the noise and the victim's belief that the noise could be reduced by another party can magnify the negative aftereffects of noise.[59] People who are affected by unrelieved barking may take revenge on the owner or even the pet. Unfortunately, appeals to owners and local law enforcement often are ineffective.[50]

Occasionally, dueling tomcats or queens in estrus contribute to noise pollution.[6] As nerve-racking as these sounds are, they rarely persist more that several nights. Losing even a few nights of healthy sleep can still have detrimental consequences, however, and should be taken seriously.

Waste

Baxter[60] reported that "an average dog can be expected to produce 0.25–1.25 L of urine and between 100 and 250 g of faeces daily." Independent of the possible transmission of parasitic diseases, the contamination of the environment by animal waste has other consequences.[61–63] There is growing concern that ground water, streams, lakes, and beaches may be contaminated with pathogenic gastrointestinal bacteria. Pet waste can promote weed and algae growth in lakes, limiting light penetration and other aquatic vegetation; oxygen levels decrease, eventually affecting fish and other aquatic life. Vegetation, including native grasses in city parks, may be affected adversely by the nitrogen content or other components of canine urine and feces.[64] Cats are notorious for using sandboxes or loose dirt in gardens and are a reservoir for Toxoplasma gondii.[65]

No one finds cat or dog feces in public places aesthetically pleasing. Private property owners are particularly incensed regarding excrement of pets that are not theirs. Perhaps this repulsion is an evolved trait to reduce contracting zoonotic diseases. Accumulative pet waste in an owner's yard can become so offensive to neighbors that some communities have enacted ordinances requiring owners to remove their pet's waste from their own yards regularly.[63] The pungent odor of intact male cat urine is repulsive to most people. Neighbors certainly do not appreciate that smell on their porches, doors, or gardens. Reeking odors emitted from a home or yard also can reduce the property value of nearby homes.

Feral and Free-Roaming Dogs and Cats

Feral, stray, and roaming owned animals contribute to all the disturbances mentioned previously and to the overpopulation problem of domestic dogs and cats, property damage, and injury to people and other animals. Loose animals also can cause car accidents, resulting in injury or death of the occupants, the animal, or both.

The impact of imported domestic animals, particularly goats, pigs, and cats, on the wildlife and biodiversity of the Galapagos is well known.[66,67] Examples of the decimation of wildlife species by dogs include the brown kiwis in New Zealand, sea turtles' eggs on Curtis Island off Queensland, Australia, and fairy penguins on Summerland Peninsula of the Phillip Island Penguin Reserve in Victoria.[6] In 1991, cats killed all reintroduced rufous hare-tailed wallabies in the Tanami desert in Australia.[6] The effect of domestic cats on wildlife in the United States continues to be studied, and the value of spay, neuter, and release (TNR) of feral cats continues to be debated.[68–72] Everyone agrees, however, that TNR programs should not be supported near wildlife areas.

The introduction or spread of contagious diseases among wildlife by domestic dogs and cats is of growing concern.[73,74] For example, feline leukemia virus has been found to cause renal spirochetosis in wild cougars.[75] It has been hypothesized that run-off containing cat feces has contributed to the increasing prevalence of *Toxoplasma gondii* in sea otters.[76] Several species of African mammals, including the lion, have been affected by canine distemper.[77,78]

Biologists and conservationists also have expressed concern regarding the release or escape of exotic or hybridized pets in the United States. Bengals and other domestic cat/small wild felid hybrids are assumed to posses better predatory behaviors and therefore be a greater threat to wildlife than the domestic cat.[79] Another concern has been hybridization of domestic dogs and wild wolves.[80] It has been argued, however, that effect of wolves cross-breeding with dogs may not have any serious consequences on the wolf populations because domestic traits that are detrimental to survival would be selected against.[81] Furthermore, dogs and wolves are so closely related that the American Society of Mammalogists classifies the dog as a subspecies of the wolf, *Canis lupus*.

Livestock owners in most communities are allowed to shoot with impunity dogs that roam onto their property. Some cities and communities prohibit the return or adoption of dogs confiscated for chasing or killing livestock, including dogs that chase chickens. Allowing pets to roam has negative consequences for livestock, owners, and the pets themselves.

Surplus of Unwanted Dogs and Cats

Unsupervised and unwanted dogs and cats eventually become the responsibility of the community.

The Human Society of the United States estimates that 3 to 4 million dogs and cats are euthanized yearly in shelters in the United States.[82] This number is a decrease from previous years.[83–85] In the 1970s the euthanasia rate was estimated to be between 13.5 and 18.6 million per year.[86] Reports pertaining to local populations in Ohio and Michigan also indicate declines during the last decade.[86,87] In the Ohio report, however, although the number of dogs euthanized decreased, that of cats increased in the period between 1996 and 2004.

In addition to a community's financial burden, mass euthanasia of animals, especially if they are healthy, takes an emotional toll on animal control personnel and veterinary staff.[88–91] Other factors also probably affect the emotional health of shelter personnel (eg, prolonged exposure to animals that seem to be unhappy and caring for animals with prolonged or lifetime sentences of confinement). Environmental enrichment of shelter animals may benefit both the animals and the emotional needs of the staff.

Companion animals may be relinquished to animal control or shelter facilities because of unplanned litters, owners' health and personal problems, illnesses or advanced geriatric conditions of the pets, and behavior problems.[24,84,92–96] In the 1930s, during the Great Depression, nearly a third of a million dogs and cats were euthanized annually in New York City alone.[85] Despite a steady decline in euthanasia rates in the past years, during the first quarter of 2008, the city of Los Angeles experienced a 30% increase in relinquished pets and a subsequent increase in the number of animals euthanized.[97] This trend coincides with the increase in loss of homes caused by foreclosures and evictions. It is becoming progressively more difficult to find rental properties or housing associations that allow pets. Past experiences with behavior problems of pets and irresponsible pet owners are reasons rental agencies or associations may ban or restrict pet ownership. It is particularly difficult to find accommodations for people who have more than one or two pets, medium-sized or large dogs, or dogs that may resemble breeds on "dangerous dog" lists.

With the intent of reducing surplus domestic dog and cat populations, many municipal and private shelters have enacted spay and neuter requirements before adoption. Some communities have enacted or proposed ordinances for mandatory spay and neuter of most dogs and cats.[98,99] These measures seem to be working.[100,101]

TNR programs have been implemented in many locations in the hope of reducing the feral cat population. It has been estimated, however, that more than 75% of cats in an area must be sterilized for the program to have any impact on the population.[102] TNR may work in niches where there are relatively few cats and little likelihood of an influx of new intact animals.

Studies have shown that education classes and pre-adoption counseling, particularly for new owners of puppies and kittens, increase owner retention rate of pets.[103,104] Although owners may seek help from books once pets exhibit problems, most owners are unwilling to pay for personal assistance in solving a problem.[105]

Animal Hoarding

Animal hoarding is a complex and underreported phenomena.[106] It is associated with self and family neglect, property damage, and animal suffering. Hoarding has four characteristic features: failure to provide minimal standards of care for the animals, lack of ability to recognize this failure, obsessive attempts to accumulate or keep a numbers of animals despite deteriorating conditions, and denial of problems with the living conditions of people and animals.[106]

Animal hoarders do not take their animals for preventative medical care regularly, but they might exhibit the following profile:[107]

Rarely bringing the same animal in twice
Generally seeking help only for traumatic or infectious events
Traveling great distances to consult with veterinarians
Seeking heroic and futile care for animals they have just found
Perfuming or bathing animals before a visit to conceal odors
Trying to persuade veterinarians to prescribe medications for animals not seen
Being unwilling or unable to say how many animals they have
Presenting pets with strong odor of urine, overgrown nails, and muscle atrophy
Continuing to display an interest in rescuing more animals, such as by checking the office bulletin board and questioning other clients

Obsessive compulsive disorders are no longer considered the appropriate model for understanding animal hoarding.[106,108] Animal hoarders are a heterogeneous group of people of all socioeconomic strata and educational levels. Animal hoarding may stem from interactions of several factors such as "disordered attachments, addictive behavior patterns, compulsive care-giving, dissociation, self-regulatory defects, and orbito-frontal dysfunction" and may require a triggering event. The complex nature of this syndrome requires individualized and interdisciplinary approaches to intervention and treatment. Simply confiscating the animals does not solve the problem. There is a high rate of recidivism. The Hoarding of Animals Research Consortium was established in 1997 and is an excellent resource for information on this topic.[106]

INJURIES RELATED TO DOG BITES

Aggression is the most common reason dogs are presented to animal behaviorists,[8,9,109] and dog bites and attacks are a worldwide problem.[110–114] It is impossible to know how many people are bitten each year by dogs or cats in the United States. Many bites go unreported, especially if inflicted by a family's own dog.[115] It also is possible that many bites are minor and are considered by owners to be a normal part of owning a pet. Bites that occur related to food, toys, or resting places often are not considered aggressive acts by the owner.

Numerous people are bitten seriously enough to prompt seeking medical care:[110] "In 2001, an estimated 300,000 persons (130 bites/100,000 humans) sustained bites severe enough to require treatment in U.S. emergency departments, with medical costs estimated at $102.4 million. In that same year, 5,892 people were hospitalized because of dog bite injuries." In the United States, approximately 18 people die each year as a result of dog-bite injuries. Posttraumatic stress disorder and residual fears can be a consequence of serious attacks.[116,117] It is recommended that victims of dog attacks be offered psychologic counseling and that parents of children who are injured also receive supportive help.

Over the years and across developed countries, the following data are fairly consistent:[110,118–122]

Children are bitten more often than adults.
Boys are bitten more often than girls.
Adults are bitten most often on the extremities.
Children often are bitten in the face.
Male dogs bite more often than female dogs.
Intact animals bite more often than neutered ones.
Dogs that are kept chained bite more often than dogs that are loose in the yard.
More bites occur in the summertime and on weekends.
The dogs usually are known to the victims.
The dogs usually are identified as German Shepherds, Chow Chows, Pit Bulls, Rottweilers, Labrador Retrievers, or as members of the terrier, working dog, herding, and non-sporting American Kennel Club dog groups.

Victims of serious dog attacks usually are very young or elderly. Fatal attacks generally involve more than one dog and occur in the absence of another person.[123]

Gershman and colleagues[119] conducted one of the few studies that included a control group in an attempt to identify factors predisposing dogs to biting. This study compared 178 dogs with one reported bite of a non–household member and 178 dogs from the same residential areas with no history of biting a non–household member. There were no significant differences between the two groups of dogs in attending obedience school, having been trained at home, regularly complying with commands to sit, stay, come, or lie down, or walking on a leash without pulling. Biting dogs were more likely to reside in homes with one or more children under 10 years of age and to be chained while in the yard. There was no significant difference in the occurrence of growling or snapping at visitors to the home between dogs that were chained and those not chained. The majority of reported bites occurred on the sidewalk, street, alley, or playground. Intact males and females were more likely to bite than their unaltered counterparts. Dogs identified as German shepherds and chows were more likely to be in the biting group, but when the owners were interviewed and asked to name the breed of their dog, if they answered "mixed breed," they were asked what breed they considered predominant, and the dog was classified accordingly.

In the last few decades several influential papers and press releases have listed breeds of dogs identified as being responsible for bites, serious injuries, and fatalities of people.[119,120,124] In an attempt to reduce harm to people and property, many landlords, housing associations, and a growing number of governments and insurance agencies have enacted breed-specific legislation that prohibits ownership or imposes constraints on the ownership of specific breeds of dogs. The validity, legality, enforceability, and effectiveness of breed-specific legislation has been questioned, however, and some regulations have been rescinded.[125–127]

Attempts to categorize dog-bite statistics by breed are handicapped by several factors. One rarely can draw conclusions about how likely a dog of a specific breed is to bite, because the population sizes of the different breeds of dogs in that locality usually are not known. When dog-bite statistics are compiled, the identity of the dog could have been assigned by anyone. Dog trainers, groomers, animal control officers, veterinary medical personnel, and victims or witnesses of dog bites often are asked to assign a breed, or predominant breed, to a dog. If a dog is a mixed breed, the identifier often is asked what purebred it looks most like, and the incident is attributed to that breed. Unless a dog is a registered purebred, owners often misidentify the breed of their own dogs.

Looks can be very deceiving, as recent ads by commercial DNA canine identification businesses have shown. A recent study found that 14 of 16 mixed-breed dogs (87.5%) identified by adoption agencies as having one or two specific breeds in their ancestry did not have these breeds confirmed by DNA analysis (V.L. Voith, unpublished data). More than 60 years ago, Scott and Fuller[128] published pictures demonstrating that the phenotypic morphology of a mixed-breed dog may not resemble either of the parents. Nonetheless, insurance company forms, animal control registration, veterinary medical and hospital records, bite reports, and surveys frequently require a "forced choice" breed identification. Subjective, visual breed identifications by a wide range of people have been collected as factual data and subsequently used to enact breed-specific legislation and to establish insurance guidelines and housing regulations.

SUMMARY

The value of companion animals to humankind is immeasurable, but there also can be negative aspects of life with animals. The annoyances and detrimental consequences of animals in society may result in legislation that restricts the enjoyment and ability of people to have companion animals. Unless people become more knowledgeable and responsible regarding care of companion animals, restrictions are likely to increase.

The small animal practitioner is in an influential position to help owners regarding the husbandry and care of their pets, which includes behavior wellness and responsible pet ownership. Intervention during office visits is an opportune time to assist owners but cannot prevent or solve all the community's problems. Knowledgeable professionals in all aspects of companion animal and human interactions are needed also.

Accurate knowledge about companion animal behavior and husbandry is essential for all ages and segments of society. Educational efforts along many avenues are necessary. Ideally, information should be infused in the school systems, from kindergarten through graduate and professional levels (including veterinary medical colleges). Television programming and public education announcements would be very beneficial. When education does not suffice, enforceable legislation is necessary to motive "irresponsible" owners to act like good citizens. Responsible pet owners welcome reasonable laws because the actions of irresponsible owners erode the benefits of everyone's pet ownership. Parental responsibility is also critical. Small children often are bitten by the good family pet that can no longer tolerate harassment, albeit often unintended by the child. Bites, often very serious, also occur when unsupervised children hit tethered dogs or enter fenced enclosures that contain dogs.

Veterinarians are respected and trusted professionals who can play pivotal roles in shaping local policies regarding animal control and promoting education pertaining to companion animal care and behavior. Veterinarians can provide input regarding design and layout of residential units and communal areas that facilitate pet ownership. In addition, veterinary education provides an excellent foundation for serving in administrative positions in agencies that formulate and set policies related to animals.

Given the large percentage of the population that has companion animals and the even greater proportion who are affected by companion animals, relatively few sociologic, anthropologic, and behavioral studies have looked at the human/companion animal interface. A societal phenomenon that affects more than 50% of the population would be well worth studying, especially because companion animals can affect the health of people in both positive and negative directions.

People and other animals can coexist beneficially and enhance each others' well being, but this relationship requires nurturing and oversight.

REFERENCES

1. Anderson RA. Pet animals and society. London: Bailliere Tindall; 1975.
2. Katcher AH, Beck AM. New perspectives on our lives with companion animals. Philadelphia: University of Pennsylvania Press; 1983.
3. Beck A, Katcher A. Between pets and people. Purdue: Pudue University Press; 1996.
4. Becker M. The healing powers of pets. New York: Hyperion; 2002.
5. Wells DL. Domestic dogs and human health: an overview. Br J Health Psychol 2007;12(1):145–56.
6. Murray RW. Urban animal problems. Animal behaviour: the TG Hungerford refresher course for veterinarians Proceedings (214). July 5–9, 1993
7. Voith VL. Clinical animal behavior. California Veterinarian 1979;28:21–5.
8. Borchelt PL, Voith VL. Aggressive behavior in dogs and cats. Compend Contin Educ 1985;7(11):949–60.
9. Bamberger M, Houpt KA. Signalment factors, comorbidity, and trends in behavior diagnoses in dogs; 1,644 cases (1991–2001). J Am Vet Med Assoc 2006;229(10):1591–601.
10. Knol BK. [Behavior problems in dogs. An inventory of the problems based on a survey conducted among Dutch veterinarians]. Tijdschr Diergeneeskd 1982; 107(17):623–32 [in Dutch].
11. Blackshaw JK. Abnormal behaviour in dogs. Aust Vet J 1988;65:393–5.

12. Takeuchi Y, Mori YA. Comparison of the behavioral profiles of purebred dogs in Japan to profiles of those in the United States and the United Kingdom. J Vet Med Sci 2006;68(8):789–96.

13. Shepherd AJ. Results of the 2006 AVMA survey of companion animal ownership in US pet-owning households. JAVMA 2008;232:695–6.

14. Westgarth C, Pinchbeck GL, Bradshaw JW, et al. Dog-human and dog-dog interactions of 260 dog-owning households in a community in Cheshire. Vet Rec 2008;162(14):436–42.

15. Voith VL. Attachment of people to companion animals. Vet Clin North Am Small Anim Pract 1985;1(2):289–95.

16. Voith VL, Wright JC, Danneman PJ. Is there a relationship between canine behavior problems and spoiling activities, anthropomorphism and obedience training? Appl Anim Behav Sci 1992;34:263–72.

17. Voith VL. Profile of 100 animal behavior cases. Mod Vet Pract 1981;62(6):483–4.

18. Tuber D, Hothersall D, Voith VL. Animal clinical psychology: a modest proposal. Am Psychol 1994;29:762–6.

19. Voith V. Attachment between people and their pets: behavior problems of pets that arise from the relationship between pets and people. In: Fogle B, editor. Interrelations between people and pets. Springfield (IL): Charles C Thomas; 1981. p. 271–94.

20. The American College of Veterinary Animal Behaviorists. Available at: www.veterinarybehavorists.org. Accessed July 26, 2008.

21. The Animal Behavior Society (ABS). Available at: www.animalbehavior.org/ABSAppliedBehavior. Accessed December 9, 2008.

22. Hetts S, Heinke ML, Estep DQ. Behavior wellness concepts for general veterinary practice. J Am Vet Med Assoc 2004;225:506–13.

23. Voith VL. Hospital policies for managing behavioral problems. California Veterinarian 2007;61(3).

24. Patronek GJ, Dodman NH. Attitudes, procedures, and delivery of behavior services by veterinarians in small animal practice. J Am Vet Med Assoc 1999;215:1606–11.

25. New J. Proactive behavior intervention strategies for the new puppy owner. Presented at the 145th Annual AVMA Meeting. New Orleans, July 18, 2008.

26. Bergman L, Hart BL, Bain M, et al. Evaluation of urine marking by cats as a model for understanding veterinary diagnostic and treatment approaches and client attitudes. J Am Vet Med Assoc 2002;221:1282–6.

27. Miller RM. Our profession's behavior problem. Vet Med 2008;342.

28. Hetts S. Pet behavior protocols: what to say, what to do, when to refer. Lakewood (CO): AAHA Press; 1999.

29. Lindsay SR. Handbook of applied dog behavior and training. Vol. 3: procedures and protocols. Ames (IA): Blackwell Publishing; 2005.

30. Landsberg G, Hunthausen W, Ackerman L. Handbook of behavior problems of the dog and cat. 2nd edition. Edinburgh (UK): Elsevier Saunders; 2003.

31. Hart BL, Hart LA, Bain MJ. Canine and feline behavior therapy. 2nd edition. Ames (IA): Blackwell Publishing; 2006.

32. Horwitz DF, Neilson JC. Blackwell's five-minute veterinary consult clinical companion: canine and feline behavior. Ames (IA): Willey-Blackwell; 2007.

33. Hetts S. Choosing a dog trainer or behavior consultant. CVMA Voice 2006;2:26.

34. AVSAB behavior professionals position statement. Available at: www.avsabonline.org. Accessed on June 25, 2008.

35. Sherman B. Animal behaviorists: who's who? Available at: www.animalbehaviorservice.com. Accessed on July 8, 2008.

36. Hetts S. What veterinarians need to know when identifying behavior referral sources. CVMA Voice 2006;2:18–26.
37. Psychology Licensing Law. Chapter 6.6 in the Business and Professions Code, the State of California. p. 20–5. Available at: www.psychboard.ca.gov/lawsregs/2008lawsregs.pdf. Accessed on July 25, 2008.
38. The American Registry of Professional Animal Scientists. Available at: www.arpas.org. Accessed July 26, 2008.
39. Certification Council for Professional Dog Trainers. Available at: www.ccpdt.org. Accessed July 26, 2008.
40. The National Association of Dog Obedience Instructors. Available at: www.nadoi.org. Accessed July 26, 2008.
41. International Association of Dog Professionals. Available at: www.dogpro.org. Accessed July 26, 2008.
42. The American Veterinary Society of Animal Behavior. Available at: http://www.avsabonline.org. Accessed December 9, 2008.
43. Overall KL. How do we obtain and disseminate accurate information? J Vet Behav:Clin Appl Res 2006;1:89–93.
44. Hetts S, Williams N, Estep DG, et al. Letter to the editor. J Vet Behav: Clin Appl Res 2007;2(3):78–9.
45. Luescher AU, Flannigan G, Mertens. The role and limitations of trainers in behavior treatment and therapy. J Vet Behav:Clin Appl Res 2007;2:26–7.
46. Cooper S. Letter to the editor. J Vet Behav:Clin Appl Res 2007;2(3):77.
47. Delta Society. Professional standards for dog trainers. Available at: www.deltasociety.org/toc.htm. Accessed July 3, 2008.
48. Bancroft R. Municipal government today: problems and complaints. In: NCL research report, America's mayors and councilmen: their problems and frustrations. League of Cities. Washington DC 1974.
49. Michaud DS, Keith SE, McMurrchy D. Noise annoyance in Canada. Noise Health 2005;7(27):39–47.
50. Mixon C. Available at: www.BarkingDogs.Net. Accessed June 25, 2008.
51. Jackson T. Is it time to ban dogs as household pet? Br Med J 2005;331:127.
52. Mixon C. The dog owner license as a solution to the dog barking and biting epidemic. Available at: BarkingDogs.net/solutions.shtml. Accessed June 25, 2008.
53. Poss JE, Bader JO. Attitudes toward companion animals among Hispanic residents of a Texas border community. J Appl Anim Welf Sci 2007;10(3):243–53.
54. Hsu Y, Severinghaus LL, Sepell JA. Dog keeping in Taiwan; its contributions to the problem of free-roaming dogs. J Appl Anim Welf Sci 2003;6(1):1–23.
55. Seligman MEP. Helplessness: on depression, development, and death. San Franciso (CA): W H Freeman and Company; 1975.
56. Randall J. Excessively barking dogs contribute to noise pollution. Aust Vet J 2003;84(4):191.
57. Senn CL, Lewin JD. Barking dogs as an environmental problem. J Am Vet Med Assoc 1975;166:1065–8.
58. Juarbe-Diaz SV. Assessment and treatment ofexcessive barking in the domestic dog. Vet Clin North Am Small Anim Pract 1997;27(3):515–32.
59. Berglund B, Lindvall T, Schwela D, editors. Guidelines for community noise. World Health Organization. Available at: www.who.int/docstore/peh/noise; 1999. Accessed June 26, 2008.
60. Baxter DN. The deleterious effects of dogs on human heath: dog-associated injuries. Community Medicine 1984;6:29–36.

61. Ram JL, Thompson B, Turner C, et al. Identification of pets and raccoons as sources of bacterial contamination of urban storm sewers using a sequence-based bacterial source tracing method. Water Res 2007;41(16):3605–14.
62. Schueler T, Holland H. The practice of watershed protection: techniques for protecting our nation's streams, lakes, rivers, and estuaries. 2000.
63. Pollution prevention fact sheet: animal waste collection. Available at: www.storm watercenter.net. Accessed June 26, 2008.
64. Mixon C. Available at: www.newaniamlcontrol.org. Accessed June 25, 2008.
65. Toxoplasmosis: epidemiology & risk factors. Available at: http://www.cdc.gov/toxoplasmosis/epi.html. Accessed July 26, 2008.
66. The impact of cats on Galapagos. Charles Darwin Research Station fact sheet. Available at: www.CharlesDarwinresearchStationFactSheet.org. Accessed June 29, 2008.
67. Guo J. The Galapagos Islands kiss their goat problem goodbye. Science 2006; 313:1567.
68. The cat debate. Available at: www.avma.org/onlnews/javma/jan04/040115a.asp. Accessed January 26, 2006.
69. Gorman S, Levy J, Pierce. A public policy toward the management of feral cats. Law Rev 2004;2(2):177–81.
70. Robertson SA. A review of feral cat control. J Feline Med Surg 2008;10(4): 366–75.
71. Foley P, Foley JE, Levy JK, et al. Analysis of the impact of trap-neuter-return programs on populations on feral cats. J Am Vet Med Assoc 2005;227(11): 1775–81.
72. Hughs KL, Slater MR, Hailer L. The effects of implementing a feral cat spay/-neuter program in a Florida county animal control service. J Appl Anim Welf Sci 2002;5(4):285–98.
73. Suzan G, Ceballos G. The role of feral mammals on wildlife infectious disease prevalence in two nature reserves within Mexico City limits. J Zoo Wildl Med 2005;26(3):479–84.
74. Riley SP, Foley J, Chomel B. Exposure to feline and canine pathogens in bobcats and gray foxes in urban and rural zones of a national park in California. J Wildl Dis 2004;40(1):11–22.
75. Jessup DA, Pettan KC, Lowenstine LJ, et al. Feline leukemia virus infection and renal spirochetosis in free-ranting cougar (*Felis concolor*). J Zoo Wildl Med 1993;24:7379.
76. Miller MA, Gardner IA, Kreuder C, et al. Coastal freshwater runoff is a risk factor for *Toxoplasmosa gondii* infection of southern sea otters (*Enhydra lutris nereis*). Int J Parasitol 2002;32:997–1006.
77. Munson L, Terio KA, Kock R, et al. Climate extremes promote fatal co-infections during canine distemper epidemics in African lions. African Wildlife 2008;3(6): e2545.
78. Leisewitz AL, Carter A, van Vuuren M, et al. Canine distemper infections, with special reference to South Africa, with a review of the literature. J S Afr Vet Assoc 2001;72(3):127–36.
79. Woodford R. Exotic cats and pet bears: biologists monitor exotic pets, captive wildlife. Alaska Fish & wildlife News 2005, August Available at: www.wildlife news.alaska.gov. Accessed June 28, 2008.
80. Andersone Z, Lucchini V, Ozoli J. Hybridisation between wolves and dogs in Latvia as documented using mitochondrial and microsatellite DNA markers. Mamm Biol 2002;67(2):79–90.

81. Porter S. Dr. Porter's rebuttal to Wisconsin Wolf Plan's section on wolfdogs. Available at: www.idir.net/~wolf2dog/porter1.htm. Accessed June 28, 2008.

82. HSUS pet overpopulation estimates. Available at: www.hsus.org/pets/issues. Accessed June 25, 2008.

83. From the Desk of Boks. U.S. shelter killing toll drops to 3.7 million dogs & cats: an analysis by Merritt Clifton. Available at: laanimalservices.blogspot.com/2007/08. 2007. Accessed June 29, 2008.

84. Steve Z, Zawistowski Z. Companion animals in society. Clifton Park (NY): Thomson Demar Learning; 2008.

85. Zawistowski S, Morris J. Population dynamics, overpopulation, and the welfare of companion animals: new insights on old and new data. J Appl Anim Welf Sci 1998;1(3):193–206.

86. Lord LK, Wittum TE, Ferketich AK, et al. Demographic trends for animal care and control agencies in Ohio from 1996–2004. JAVMA 2006;229:48–54.

87. Bartlett PC, Bartlett A, Walshaw S, et al. Rates of euthanasia and adoption for dogs and cats in Michigan animal shelters. J Appl Anim Welf Sci 2005;8:97–104.

88. Rowan A. Shelters and pet overpopulation: a statistical black hole. Anthrozoos 1992;5:140–3.

89. White DJ, Shawhan R. Emotional responses of animal shelter workers to euthanasia. J Am Vet Med Assoc 1996;208:846–9.

90. Rogelberg SG, DiGiacomo N, Reeve CL, et al. What shelters can do about euthanasia-related stress: an examination of recommendations from those on the front line. J Appl Anim Welf Sci 2007;10(4):331–47.

91. Rogelberg SG, Reeve CL, Spitzmuller C, et al. Impact of euthanasia rates, euthanasia practices, and human resource practices on employee turnover in animal shelters. J Am Vet Assoc 2007;230(5):713–9.

92. Patronek GL, Glickman LT, Beck AM, et al. Risk factors for relinquishment of dogs to an animal shelter. J Am Vet Assoc 1996;209(3):572–81.

93. Shore ER. Returning a recently adopted companion animal; adopters' reasons for and reactions to the failed adoption experience. J Appl Anim Welf Sci 2005;8(3):187–98.

94. Salman MD, Hutchiinson J, Ruch-Gallie R, et al. Behavioral reasons for relinquishment of dogs and cats to 12 shelters. J Appl Anim Welf Sci 2000;3(20):93–106.

95. Scarlett JM, Slaman MD, New JG, et al. Reasons for relinquishment of companion animals in U.S. shelters: selected health and personal issues. J Appl Ani Welf Sci 1999;2(1):41–57.

96. New JC Jr, Salman MD, Scarlett JM, et al. Characteristics of dogs and cats and those relinquishing them to 12 U.S. animal shelters. J Appl Ani Welf Sci 1999;2(2):83–97.

97. From the Desk of Ed Boks. Breaking down the numbers April 20, 2008. Available at: www.laanimalservices.blogspot.com. Accessed July 9, 2008.

98. Spay/neutered required for cats and dogs in Los Angeles City. Available at: www.laanimalservices.com. Accessed July 9 2008.

99. Goodyear C. Supervisors vote to require neutering of pit bulls, mixes in Contra Costa, Board votes to bar felons from owning big dogs. San Francisco Chronicle 2005. Available at: www.sfgate.com. Accessed July 9, 2008.

100. Lieberman LL. A case for neutering pups and kittens at two months of age. J Am Vet Med Assoc 1987;191:518–21.

101. Lagos MSF. Sterilization law successful in reducing pit bull population. San Francisco Chronicle 2007. Available at: www.sfisonline.com. Accessed July 9, 2008.

102. Andersen MC, Martin BJ, Roemer GW. Use of matrix population models to estimate the efficacy of euthanasia versus trap-neuter-return for management of free roaming cats. JAVMA 2004;225(12):1871–6.
103. Duxbury MM, Jackson JA, Line SW, et al. Evaluation of association between retention in the home and attendance at puppy socialization classes. J Am Vet Assoc 2003;223(1):61–6.
104. Herron ME, Lord LK, Hill LN, et al. Effects of preadoption counseling for owners on house-training success among dogs acquire from shelters. J Am Vet Assoc 2007;231(4):558–62.
105. Shore ER, Burdsal C, Douglas DK. Pet owner's views of pet behavior problems and willingness to consult experts for assistance. J Appl Anim Welf Sci 2008;11:63–73.
106. Animal hoarding: structuring interdisciplinary responses to help people, animals and communities at risk. Patronek GJ, Loar L, Nathanson JN, eds. 2006 Hoarding of Animals Research Consortium. Available at: www. Hoarding of Animals Research Consortium.
107. Patronek G. Tips for identifying animal hoarders. JAVMA 2002;221(8):1088–9.
108. Patronek G. Animal hoarding: what caseworkers need to know. Animal Rescue League of Boston Mass Housing Community Services Conference 2007. Animal Rescue League of Boston.
109. Beaver BV. Clinical classification of canine aggression. Appl Anim Ethol 1983;10:35–43.
110. Shuler CM, DeBess EE, Lapidus JA, et al. Canine and human factors related to dog bite injuries. J Am Vet Assoc 2008;232(4):542–6.
111. Centers for Disease Control and Prevention (CDC). Nonfatal dog bite-related injuries treated in hospital emergency departments—United States, 2001. MMWR Morb Mortal Wkly Rep 2003;52(26):605–10.
112. MacBean CE, Taylor DM, Ashby K. Animal and human bite injuries in Victoria, 1998–2004. Med J Aust 2007;186(1):38–40.
113. Dwyer JP, Douglas TS, van As AB. Dog bite injuries in children—a review of data from a South African paediatric trauma unit. S Afr Med J 2007;97(8):597–600.
114. Rosado B, Garcia-Belenguer S, Leon M, et al. A comprehensive study of dog bites in Spain, 1995–2004. Vet J 2008 [E pub ahead of print].
115. Beck AM, Jones BA. Unreported dog bites in children. Public Health Rep 1985;100:315–21.
116. Rossman BB, Bingham RD, Emde RN. Symptomatology and adaptive functioning for children exposed to normative stressors, dog attack, and parental violence. J Am Acad Child Adolesc Psychiatry 1997;36(8):1089–97.
117. De Keuster T, Lamoureux J, Kahn A. Epidemiology of dog bites: a Belgian experience of canine behaviour and public health concerns. Vet J 2006;172(3):482–7.
118. Clifton M. Dog attack deaths and maimings, U.S. & Canada, September 1982 to November 13, 2006. Animal People 2007.
119. Gershman KA, Sacks JJ, Wright JC. Which dogs bite? A case-control study of risk factors. Pediatrics 1994;93:913–6.
120. Sacks JJ, Sinclair L, Gilchrist J, et al. Breeds of dogs involved in fatal human attacks in the United States between 1979 and 1998. JAVMA 2000;217:836–40.
121. Wright JC. Severe attacks by dogs: characteristics of the dogs, the victims, and the attack settings. Public Health Rep 1985;100:55–61.
122. Thompson PG. The public health impact of dog attacks in a major Australian city. Med J Aust 1997;167(3):129–32.

123. Borchelt PL, et al. Attacks by packs of dogs involving predation on human beings. Public Health Rep 1983;98:57–65.
124. Sacks JJ, Sattin RW, Bonzo SE. Dog-bite related fatalities from 1979 through 1988. JAMA 1989;262:1489–92.
125. Bandow JH. Will breed-specific legislation reduce dog bites? Can Vet J 1996; 37:478–83.
126. Ledger RA, Orihel JS, Clarke N, et al. Breed specific legislation: considerations for evaluating its effectiveness and recommendations for alternatives. Can Vet J 2005;46:735–43.
127. Delise K. The pit bull placebo. Ramsey (NJ): Anubis Publishing; 2007.
128. Scott JP, Fuller JL. Genetics and the social behavior of the dog. Chicago: The University of Chicago Press; 1965.

Emergency Management During Disasters for Small Animal Practitioners

Helen T. Engelke, BVSc, MPVM, MRCVS

KEYWORDS

- Disaster preparedness • Small animal clinician
- Small animal practitioner • Emergency management
- Veterinary issues in disasters

To small animal practitioners addressing the immediate clinical concerns of their patients, the relevance of emergency management and disaster preparedness may not be readily apparent. But given the potential for unforeseen events, it is worthwhile to consider one's level of personal preparedness, the preparedness of the practice facilities, and the safety of colleagues, staff and co-workers. It also is important to acquaint oneself with the relevant governmental agencies, community stakeholders, and volunteer opportunities before an event occurs.

Familiarity with the principles of emergency management enables one to respond professionally during an event and also provides peace of mind. It is useful to reflect on the Veterinarian's Oath that states a commitment "to the benefit of society."[1] Accordingly, veterinarians' responsibilities extend beyond the health of the animals in their care to include safeguarding the health of humans. As health professionals, with responsibilities to the physical, mental, and social well being of the people in the community, it is important for veterinarians to recognize how these facets of human well being are affected by the plight of animals during disasters.

This article acquaints the small animal practitioner with principles of emergency management during a disaster, including the organizational structure of emergency management and the emergency management cycle. Specific activities that small animal clinicians might engage in with regards to disaster mitigation, preparedness, response, and recovery are discussed. In addition, opportunities for training and community involvement for the small animal veterinarian are highlighted.

College of Veterinary Medicine, Western University of Health Sciences, 309 E Second Street, Pomona, CA 91766, USA
E-mail address: hengelke@westernu.edu

Vet Clin Small Anim 39 (2009) 347–358
doi:10.1016/j.cvsm.2008.10.013
0195-5616/08/$ – see front matter © 2009 Elsevier Inc. All rights reserved.

vetsmall.theclinics.com

ORGANIZATIONAL STRUCTURE

The old adage that "all disasters are local" is still relevant to modern emergency management. Depending on the magnitude of a disaster, however, varying levels of involvement by government agencies and nonprofit groups may be required. An understanding of the organizational structure under which the emergency management system operates allows those involved to function more efficiently, with minimal conflict and redundancy.

Local Government

Most towns and cities within the United States have an Office of Emergency Management that can activate Emergency Operations Centers to make operational decisions during emergencies. The manpower and budgetary allocations of these offices generally correlate with the population size of the city. Although small rural communities may lack an Office of Emergency Management, usually at least one individual within the municipal government is assigned the tasks of emergency manager.

Each county also has an Office of Emergency Management, which has the statutory authority to manage emergency events. Its responsibilities include planning and coordination, operations, training, public education, and resource acquisition. Because many city Offices of Emergency Management may coexist within a county's jurisdiction, there may be mutual aid agreements and memoranda of understanding to manage better the multijurisdictional distribution of resources.

For veterinarians working in and serving local communities, an important first step is to locate the local Office of Emergency Management and become familiar with its internal organizational structure and points of contact before an event occurs. The events following Hurricane Katrina enhanced the public's awareness of animal issues related to disasters. The input of professional veterinarians at the local level is still limited, however, and most municipalities welcome insight and advice from those who have expertise in animal issues. Their planning, preparedness, response, and recovery efforts are enhanced by collaboration with local veterinarians, veterinary technicians, and animal handlers.

State Government

Although the first level of response to any event is the responsibility of the local agency, the scope of an event may overwhelm local resources rapidly. At this time the governor of the state may proclaim a disaster in affected counties, allowing state resources (human, physical, and/or financial) to flow to these counties. The governor also may deploy National Guard troops to assist in emergency management.

State Offices of Emergency Management often have regional offices throughout the state that provide support to local governments under the invitation of the local chief executive officer. These regional offices also monitor events and advise the state governor if federal assistance is warranted. If so, the governor can request a major disaster declaration from the President. Such requests always are initiated by the governor.

Federal Government

A number of federal departments carry out roles related to disasters (eg, the Department of Agriculture [USDA], the Department of Health and Human Services, which includes the Centers for Disease Control and Prevention and Food and Drug Administration, and the Department of Defense). The agency with the most direct involvement is the Department of Homeland Security's Federal Emergency Management Agency (FEMA). FEMA was formed following an executive order of President Carter in 1979.[2] Its statutory authority is the Robert T. Stafford Disaster Relief and Emergency Assistance Act, PL 100-707.[3] In March 2003, FEMA was integrated into the Department of Homeland Security, which was formed in response to the terrorist attacks on September 11, 2001.[3] The primary mission of FEMA is

> to reduce the loss of life and property and protect the Nation from all hazards, including natural disasters, acts of terrorism, and other man-made disasters, by leading and supporting the Nation in a risk-based, comprehensive emergency management system of preparedness, protection, response and recovery and mitigation.[3]

The federal government's involvement in emergency management has been expanded by the possibility of a bioterrorism event. The primary responding agency is determined by the type of event. If there were an intentional or unintentional introduction of a foreign animal disease, the USDA's Animal Plant Health Inspection Service would take the lead. If the incident involved meat or poultry, the USDA's Food Safety Inspection Service would be responsible. If the event targeted any other food, it would fall under the purview of the Food and Drug Administration. Any event affecting human health also would be investigated by the Centers for Disease Control and Prevention.

American Indian and Alaska Native Tribal Governments

American Indian and Alaska Native tribal governments coexist within the United States with the benefits and rights of sovereign nations. As such, many have their own emergency management systems that work with FEMA and state and local agencies. These collaborations stand to provide mutual benefits to all involved.

Volunteer Organizations Active in Disasters

Nonprofit private agencies offer critical support through all aspects of an emergency event and are an essential part of the emergency management community. The American Red Cross and the Salvation Army are the primary agencies dealing with human concerns during a disaster. In addition, there now is a cadre of organizations whose primary focus relates to animal issues during disasters.

One of the major concerns raised following Hurricane Katrina was how to maximize the resources of multiple nonprofit agencies. One result was the formation of the National Animal Rescue and Sheltering Coalition (NARSC). NARSC brings together major national animal welfare groups bimonthly to enhance the overall response of the nonprofit agencies to animal issues during disasters.[4] Members of NARSC include the American Society for the Prevention of Cruelty to Animals, the American Humane Association, Best Friends Animal Society, Code 3 Associates, the Humane Society of the United States, the International Fund for Animal Welfare, the National Animal Control Association, the United Animal Nations/Emergency Animal Rescue Services, and the Society of Animal Welfare Administrators. Its mission is "To identify, prioritize and find collaborative solutions to major human-animal emergency issues."[5]

THE EMERGENCY MANAGEMENT CYCLE

With the formation of FEMA, the need for an all-hazards approach[6] to potential threats to life, rather than distinct plans for separate incidents, became apparent. Although each disaster is unique, common strategies can be used to manage them. An emergency cycle consisting of four management phases—mitigation, preparedness, response, and recovery—can be used to describe any event. Regardless of whether an event is natural (ie, catastrophic earthquake, flood, or hurricane) or intentional, veterinarians can be involved and make important contributions in each of these phases.

Phase 1: Mitigation

FEMA defines mitigation as "the effort to reduce loss of life and property by lessening the impact of disasters."[7] In a veterinary practice setting mitigation can be implemented in a number of ways. For instance, if a small animal practice is located in a community susceptible to flooding, purchasing adequate flood insurance and adequately anchoring any mobile buildings on the premises would be examples of mitigating activities. Similarly, for those in tornado-susceptible locations, having a designated tornado shelter and replacing windows with nonshattering glass would be mitigating activities.

Every practice, even those not located in extreme weather zones, hurricane belts, or earthquake zones, is vulnerable to disasters. Incidents such as industrial accidents or accidents involving transportation of hazardous material can occur almost anywhere. In 1996, a small town in rural Wisconsin was evacuated following the derailment of a passing freight train and ensuing fire. Residents had to evacuate quickly, and many left without their pets.[8] Incidents also can be small in scale, such as the evacuation of a veterinary practice following a vehicle accident that compromises the integrity of the building. Although every possible event cannot be foreseen, the important point is to get started by designating some time and resources to the topic of mitigation in the practice setting.

Veterinarians also have an ethical responsibility to advise clients of mitigation activities to consider for their pets, such as providing adequate identification by microchipping or tags and keeping current photographs of their pets in a secure location. This topic can be integrated into the pet's routine veterinary care, such as during a wellness visit. After Katrina, pet owners experienced significant emotional distress when many could not adequately prove ownership of their pets.

Phase 2: Preparedness

Preparedness activities include determining risk, planning for an emergency, assembling supplies and human resources, and practicing the implementation of those plans by training and conducting disaster drills. Such preparation activities serve to minimize the emotional and financial consequences of a disaster.

Federal preparedness
Since October 2001, following the events of September 11, the President's homeland security policies have been recorded in Homeland Security Presidential Directives (HSPDs).[9] More than 20 HSPDs have been released.

HSPD[8] focuses on preparedness. Released in December 2003, it

establishes policies to strengthen the preparedness of the United States to prevent and respond to threatened or actual domestic terrorist attacks, major disasters and other emergencies by requiring a national domestic all hazards preparedness goal, establishing mechanisms for improved delivery of federal preparedness assistance to state and local governments and outlining actions to strengthen preparedness capabilities of federal, state and local entities.[10]

HSPD[8] requires that all federal departments and agencies, not just the Department of Homeland Security and FEMA, establish preparedness goals by assessing priorities, identifying capabilities, and strengthening delivery of assistance to the state and local agencies they serve.

As part of the preparedness plan, the federal government published the National Preparedness Guidelines in September 2007.[11] The guidelines include 15 national planning scenarios that identify events of high consequence, including events of natural origin and deliberate terrorist acts. Scenarios that are of particular relevance to veterinarians include an aerosol anthrax attack, pandemic influenza, plague, the introduction of a foreign animal disease, and food contamination. The 15 scenarios provide the basis for all federal planning, training exercises, and grant distribution to other agencies for disaster preparation.

To prevent and respond to any of these scenarios, 1600 tasks (the Universal Task list) were identified along with 37 specific capabilities (the Target Capabilities list). These capabilities are ones that communities, the private sector, and all levels of government need to possess to respond to a disaster. One such capability is "Animal Disease Emergency Support." This capability expects that the United States would be prepared to respond adequately to any "incident that would result in the disruption of industries related to US livestock, other domestic animals (including companion animals) and wildlife and or endanger the food supply, public health and domestic and international trade."[12] Fulfillment of this capability expects that foreign animal diseases would be prevented from entering the United States, but if one did gain entry, the disease would be detected early, thereby minimizing the consequences to agriculture.

Involvement of all stakeholders is vital to the successful implementation of the National Preparedness Guidelines. This collaboration involves multiple parties, such as the USDA's Animal Plant Health Inspection Service (APHIS) and the Food Safety Inspection Service; the Centers for Disease Control and Prevention; state, county, and city emergency operations centers; and local responders such as veterinarians, animal health technicians, veterinary epidemiologists, animal welfare specialists, laboratory technicians, and wildlife experts.

State preparedness

State departments of agriculture always have had responsibility for preparedness activities for livestock. Following the events of Hurricane Katrina, however, it was recognized that insufficient emphasis had been placed on planning for companion animals in disasters. The Pets Evacuation and Transportation Standards (PETS) Act of 2006 was enacted in part to correct these deficiencies. The PETS Act requires that state and local emergency operational plans "take into account the needs of individuals with household pets and service animals before, during and following a major disaster or emergency."[13] It also budgets for federal financial assistance to state and local agencies for animal preparedness purposes. State departments of agriculture have taken the lead in preparedness activities related to companion animals. Although the PETS Act has provided the impetus for many states to develop companion animal preparedness plans, it is limited in scope and does not delineate which specifics the plans should include, nor does it provide funding for implementing plans during a real event.

Many state departments of agriculture have acted as conduits, bringing together county and local animal agencies, nonprofit volunteer agencies, local veterinarians, and other animal stakeholders to develop regional plans for evacuation and shelter of companion animals. The public health issue of persons potentially endangering their own safety rather than evacuating without their pets or refusing to evacuate to a shelter that does not accommodate companion animals has prompted many states to develop plans that will serve the needs of their constituents better in the event of a disaster.

A major component of many state preparedness activities includes statewide exercises. One such program is the California Golden Guardian exercise, which annually simulates an event such as a catastrophic earthquake.[14] Such simulations provide an excellent method for veterinarians to assess their preparedness for an event. The California Department of Agriculture, through its California Animal Emergency Response System, actively encourages the participation of the veterinary community in this statewide initiative.

Clinic preparedness

Although most veterinary practices post a building evacuation plan in case of fire, equal consideration should be given to a written disaster preparedness plan. That plan should consider the following issues.

Sheltering on-site If an event were to occur that required every animal and human to remain on the premises, sufficient food and water would be needed for all. Many plans recommend having resources for a 72-hour period, but this duration should be considered the absolute minimum. In addition, a system should be in place to notify clients as to the status of their animals.

Evacuation plan Once an evacuation plan is in place, it needs to be practiced regularly. These drills should be solution based, with the focus on identifying insufficiencies and taking corrective action. For instance, a fire officer or an emergency services worker could come to the practice and state that the practice has 15 minutes to evacuate the premises. A drill would help identify whether the practice has everything in place to facilitate such an event, such as sufficient pet carriers and leashes, adequate staff training, and specific plans for animals in intensive care. Although the priority in any disaster is saving human life, a good evacuation plan can prevent or minimize loss of life to the animals in the veterinarian's care.

Consideration also should be given to selection of the site to which the practice evacuates. Prewritten memoranda of understanding with both local and regional veterinary practices would allow efficient relocation of animals from one practice to another. Instituting telephone trees with veterinary colleagues, in which each individual is preassigned to communicate with only two or three other individuals, can help ensure a timely and efficient flow of information.

Disaster kit A veterinary clinic probably will have most of the medical supplies that a disaster kit requires. In addition, it is important to assemble such items as heavy-duty gloves, a crow bar, a hammer, battery-operated or hand-cranked flash lights and radio, a telephone that can operate without electricity, and sufficient potable water and food. The disaster kit should be identified to all staff and placed in an accessible location.

Employee training Training is an essential part of a good preparedness plan. A variety of options are available for training veterinarians and their employees in the field of emergency management. FEMA's Emergency Management Institute has an independent study program offering free online courses.[15] The courses offered support the mission areas identified by the National Preparedness Goal and include Incident Management, Operational Planning, Disaster Logistics, Emergency Communications, Service to Disaster Victims, Continuity Programs, Public Disaster Communications, Integrated Preparedness, and Hazard Mitigation.[15] The completion of many of these FEMA courses serves as the minimum requirement for serving as a disaster responder in both governmental and nonprofit agencies. Persons interested in serving as disaster responders should check with the agency they are most likely to work with to determine which FEMA courses are recommended.

FEMA also has a Center for Domestic Preparedness whose mission is "to operate a federal training center for the delivery of high quality comprehensive preparedness training programs for the nation's emergency responders."[16]

One course offered through the Center that may be of particular interest to veterinarians, veterinary technicians, and animal care workers is a 4-day Weapons of Mass Destruction Agricultural Emergency Responder training course.[17]

Many volunteer organizations active in disasters such as the Humane Society of the United States,[18] the United Animal Nations/Emergency Animal Rescue Services,[19] and American Humane[20] also offer training courses specifically for persons with animal expertise. These courses are of variable length and are tailored to differing target audiences.

For persons who want a more in-depth exposure to the field, many university Masters of Public Health programs offer an emphasis on emergency management, biosecurity, and disaster preparedness. Certification programs in emergency management also are available and offer coursework that can be completed in less time than needed for a degree program.

Numerous training programs are available to meet all levels of interest and commitment. State departments of agriculture and state public health veterinarians can prove an excellent resource in identifying suitable training courses in a particular area. The American Veterinary Medical Association also provides a comprehensive list of training opportunities.[21]

Pet-owner preparedness

Veterinarians are a primary resource for clients regarding pet disaster preparedness. Such information could be integrated into a routine wellness visit and included in posters, pamphlets, and videos available in the waiting areas and examination rooms. This information should include a list of things to include in an evacuation kit, such as food, water, medications, medical records, first aid supplies, collars, identification tags, leashes, pet carriers, litter boxes, and pictures of pets with owners as extra proof of ownership. Pets also will require basic command training and familiarization with the carrier before any disaster. Clients should include pets in the family evacuation plans; these plans should include telephone numbers for pet-friendly hotels and regional veterinarians. In addition, if the pet must be left at home, advance planning is needed to determine the best room in which to leave the pet, to ensure adequate food and water, and to notify responders that a pet is on the premises. Owners vary considerably in their level of preparedness for themselves and their pets, but at least the veterinarian can help ensure that the pets are not overlooked.

A thorough discussion of the components of a pet-owner disaster preparedness plan is beyond the scope of this article, but veterinarians can obtain client educational materials for their practice from the Department of Homeland Security's "Ready Now" campaign,[22] the American Veterinary Medical Association,[23] and the Humane Society of the United States.[24] Clients also can be directed to the online resources which these groups provide regarding disaster planning for pets. In addition, consultation with organizations such as the American Red Cross can provide detailed information on preparedness for clients as well as clinic staff.[25]

Phase 3: Response

The third phase of the emergency management cycle, response, occurs both during and after the disaster. Response includes all activities involved in preserving human and animal lives, such as rescuing injured individuals and animals, executing evacuation plans, providing medical and veterinary care, providing food, shelter, and counseling to those displaced, and re-establishing civic order for the protection of all.

Administrative structure

The National Incident Management System Major incidents may require responders to draw quickly upon multiple disciplines and multiple jurisdictions. The National Incident Management System (NIMS) was established following Homeland Security Presidential Directive 5 in February 2003. The directive's purpose is "To enhance the ability of the United States to manage domestic incidents by establishing a single, comprehensive, national incident management system."[26]

The NIMS facilitates coordination between responders from federal, state, and local government agencies, nonprofit agencies, and volunteer groups. It works at two levels, using the Incident Command System (ICS) and the Multiagency Coordination System (MACS) to manage the response to an event.

The Incident Command System The ICS is an on-scene, standardized management system designed to dictate the immediate response to all types of disasters. The system had seen success in the firefighting community before its inclusion in NIMS.28 It uses common terminology to facilitate efficient communication among multiple individuals from various agencies. It also is flexible enough to be used in any kind of incident.

The system recognizes specific activities that occur in any disaster event and assigns an individual with responsibility to those activities. These designations are

- The Incident Commander, who assumes overall leadership for the event
- The Command Staff, comprised of a safety officer, who is responsible for the safety of the responders; a liaison officer, who acts as a point of contact for all supporting agencies; and a public information officer, who is tasked with providing all suitable and necessary information to the public following consultation with the incident commander and general staff.[27]
- The General Staff, comprised of four section chiefs: the operations section chief, the planning sections chief, the logistics section chief, and the finance section chief. As an incident expands, each of these four sections may expand to include its own branches, divisions, or groups.[27]

Depending on the scope of the event and the degree of adherence to the ICS principles, any number of responders can work in concert at a site to manage the incident effectively. The system is weakened when responders are unfamiliar with its structure. Therefore, anyone wanting to work as a first responder, including veterinarians, should familiarize themselves with ICS through such offerings as the free on-line course available through FEMA's Emergency Management Institute.[28]

Multiagency Coordination Systems The other operational component of NIMS is the MACS. As the name suggests, MACS are established to coordinate better facilities, equipment, personnel, procedures, and communications for all of the responding agencies from multiple jurisdictions during an event. For example, if a flood were to occur in a given county, the MACS might involve multiple city emergency operations centers within that county.[29]

Veterinary involvement in response

Veterinarians and veterinary technicians can offer their expertise in response to a disaster in a number of ways and through a variety of agencies. Local and state health department officials and state department of agriculture veterinarians can be a good resource for identifying opportunities at the local level. Some potential opportunities for veterinary involvement are discussed here.

National Veterinary Response Team The National Veterinary Response Team (NVRT) is comprised of veterinarians, animal health technicians, epidemiologists, and other public health professionals who volunteer to be activated during a disaster. The program is part of the National Disaster Medical System of the Department of Health and Human Services. Deployed team members are compensated for their time, because the NVRT is a fully supported federal program. The NVRT responsibilities include[30]

- Assessing the veterinary medical needs of the community
- Medical treatment and stabilization of animals
- Animal disease surveillance
- Zoonotic disease surveillance and public health assessments
- Technical assistance to assure food safety and water quality
- Hazard mitigation
- Care and support of animals certified as official responders to a disaster or emergency

The National Animal Health Emergency Response Corps The USDA, APHIS established the National Animal Health Emergency Response Corps (NAHERC) in 2001 to provide assistance in the event of a major outbreak of a foreign animal disease.[31] In the event of an outbreak, APHIS would call on NAHERC members, who are veterinarians and veterinary students, to be activated as federal employees of USDA, APHIS.[32] NAHERC members assisted with the exotic Newcastle disease outbreak in California in 2003 and contributed to the efforts to eradicate foot and mouth disease in the United Kingdom in 2001.[31]

State animal response teams Many individual states also have animal response teams consisting of veterinarians and other animal stakeholders. The administration of these teams varies from state to state, with some state teams operating through state veterinarians and others through state veterinary medical associations.[31] Officials at state and local health departments and state departments of agriculture can assist veterinary practitioners with identifying opportunities for involvement.

Volunteer Organizations Active in Disasters Nonprofit agencies also recruit volunteers to serve on animal response teams. The Humane Society of the United States operates the National Disaster Animal Response Team. Internal training is offered to volunteers, who also are required to complete FEMA independent study coursework.[33] United Animal Nations uses its Emergency Animal Rescue Services to shelter and care for animals displaced during disasters and has more than 4000 volunteers.[34] American Humane's Red Star Animal Emergency Services also functions with the assistance of volunteers.[35] Many other nonprofit agencies, supported by volunteer animal response teams, exist in local communities.

Clinic response Although opportunities abound for individual veterinarians to assist others during a disaster, situations may arise in which a veterinary clinic becomes involved as a temporary shelter site during an emergency. This function should be assumed only in coordination with the local emergency operations center to be sure that issues of liability insurance and compensation are addressed. Reimbursements may be available for costs relating to evacuations and sheltering, although this reimbursement currently is limited to federally declared disasters and for shelters operating under the umbrella of the local emergency operations centers.[36]

In the event of a major disaster, it is common for individuals to volunteer their services. Persons may just show up at a clinic wanting to assist. Sometimes a distinction is made between spontaneous volunteers who come forward and ask to help, such as at a temporary shelter, versus convergent volunteers who turn up at a site and just start to help, such as following a catastrophic earthquake. In either case it is important to encourage such volunteers to operate under the umbrella of the local emergency operations center. Many states have disaster service worker programs allowing individuals to be sworn in and to function with some protection against liability. Although most disaster service worker programs require prior training, en masse swearing in ceremonies can take place as part of a response to a major event.

Phase 4: Recovery

The fourth phase of the emergency management cycle is recovery from the disaster. This phase includes all the postdisaster activities that help the affected community return to normal. Typically, but not always, the speed and expense of the recovery depends on the magnitude of the event. A complex array of social, geopolitical, and economic factors dictate the way a community recovers from a disaster.

The social disruption to the community following a disaster may be overwhelming. Governmental agencies may have to deal with disruptions to their infrastructure, transportation, and utilities. Individuals may be searching for displaced family members or pets, dealing with the loss of a home and forced relocation, filing insurance claims, coping with the disruption to employment and loss of income, and cleaning up their property.

It is important for veterinarians to recognize the psychologic impact disasters have on clients. The stress resulting from the many disruptions to everyday life may explain why the incidence of pet abandonment increases following a disaster. Practitioners should be aware that extensions to time frames after which an animal is considered abandoned are often included in emergency regulations.

Conversely the human–animal bond can be important in sustaining pet owners through periods of undue stress. Strong emotional attachments to pets can be expected. Veterinary roles following a disaster event may expand to include being a confidant, a lay counselor, a community advocate, and even a community activist.

Veterinarians in the affected area may see a rise in animals presenting with specific health issues relating to the disaster. An increase in the incidence of respiratory, dermatologic, and infectious disease may occur following a flood. Similarly, an increase in the incidence of traumatic injuries might be anticipated after an earthquake or hurricane, as animals come in contact with debris. Depending on the type of disaster, animals also may be seen with exposures to hazardous materials or suffering smoke inhalation. Veterinarians also may note a rise in owners presenting with complaints of behavioral changes in their pets, such as increased aggression, barking without reason, or being unexpectedly withdrawn, behaviors that could indicate a diagnosis of posttraumatic stress disorder.[37]

The recovery phase of the cycle also involves documenting and reviewing activities relating to the disaster. Developing "after action reports," evaluating what worked and what did not, and determining what improvements can be made ultimately assists in better mitigation and preparedness for future events.

SUMMARY

Having an understanding of the key components of emergency management, the organizational structure, and the emergency management cycle are important steps in understanding how veterinarians can contribute to all aspects of mitigation, preparedness, response, and recovery. Before an event it also is important to identify the key persons one needs to work with, such as local emergency operations officials and animal response team coordinators. There are many opportunities for veterinarians to receive disaster training and to get involved before an event. Such veterinary participation ultimately has a positive impact on pets, the veterinarian's clients, and the entire community.

REFERENCES

1. American Veterinary Medical Association. Veterinarians oath. About the AVMA. Available at: http://www.avma.org/about_ avma/whoweare/default.asp. Accessed June 16, 2008.
2. Federal Emergency Management Agency. Executive order 12127. FEMA history. Available at: http://www.fema.gov/about/history.shtm. Accessed June 17, 2008.
3. Federal Emergency Management Agency. About FEMA. Available at: http://www.fema.gov/about/index.shtm. Accessed June 17, 2008.
4. Ballard P. How Katrina galvanized disaster response for animals. Available at: http://hsus.org/hsus_field/hsus_disaster_center_/disasters_press_room/katrina_anniversary/katrina_disaster_services.html. August 27, 2007. Accessed June 16, 2008.
5. National Animal Control Association. Disaster database. Available at: http://nacanet.org/disasterdatabase.html. Accessed June 18, 2008.
6. Emergency Management Institute. Available at: http://emilms.fema.gov/IS Federal 10/FEMA_IS/IS10/index.htm. Accessed June 16, 2008.
7. Federal Emergency Management Agency. FEMA mitigation. Available at: http://fema.gov/government/mitigation.shtm. Accessed June 18, 2008.
8. Grendahl LG. Wisconsin train derailment turns veterinarians into heroes. J Am Vet Med Assoc 1996;208(10):1611–2.
9. The White House. Homeland Security Presidential Directive–1. Available at: http://www.whitehouse.gov/news/releases/2001/10/print/20011030-1.html. Accessed June 27, 2008.
10. Homeland Security Presidential Directive–8. Available at: http://www.whitehouse.gov/news/releases/2003/12/print/20031217-6.html. Accessed June 27, 2008.
11. US Department of Homeland Security. National Preparedness Guidelines September 2007. Available at: http://www.fema.gov/pdf/government/npg.pdf. Accessed December 19, 2008.
12. US Department of Homeland Security. Target capabilities list—a companion to the National Preparedness Guidelines. US Department of Homeland Security. Available at: http://www.fema.gov/pdf/government/training/tcl.pdf. Accessed December 19, 2008.
13. Pets Evacuation and Transportation Standards Act of 2006 Public Law 109–308. 109th Congress. Available at: http://frwebgate.access.gpo/cgi_bin/getdoc.cgi?dbname=109_cong_public_laws&docid=f:publ307.109.pdf. Accessed December 19, 2008.
14. California Office of Emergency Services. State of California exercise program. Available at: http://www.oes.ca.gov/WebPage/oeswebsite.nsf/Content/70614BCE9D2EB927882574D007003BC?OpenDocument. Accessed July 25, 2008.
15. Emergency Management Institute. Independent study program courses. Available at: http://training.fema.gov/IS/crslist.asp. Accessed June 28, 2008.
16. Center for Domestic Preparedness. About the Center for Domestic Preparedness. Available at: https://cdp.dhs.gov/about.html. Accessed June 16, 2008.
17. Center for Domestic Preparedness. Center for Domestic Preparedness course details. Available at: https://cdp.dhs.gov/resident/agert.html. Accessed June 16, 2008.

18. The Humane Society of the United States. Disaster training program for 2008. Available at: http://www.hsus.org/hsus_field/hsus_disaster_center_/disaster_training_dates_2007.html. Accessed July 25, 2008.

19. United Animal Nations/Emergency Animal Rescue Services. Volunteer training. Available at: http://www.uan.org/index.cfm?navid=35. Accessed July 25, 2008.

20. American Humane Society. AES basic training. Available at: http://www.americanhumane.org/site/PageServer?pagename=ev_professionals_aes_training. Accessed July 25, 2008.

21. The American Veterinary Medical Association. Animal health disaster training. Available at: http://www.avma.org/disaster/training.asp. Accessed July 25, 2008.

22. Preparing your pets for emergencies makes sense. Get ready now. [brochure]. Available at: http://www.ready.gov/america/_downloads/pets.pdf. Accessed June 28, 2008.

23. Lovern CS. Saving the whole family. [brochure]. Available at: http://www.avma.org/disaster/saving_family_brochure.pdf. Accessed June 28, 2008.

24. The Humane Society of the United States. Disaster preparedness for pets. Available at: http://www.hsus.org/hsus_field/hsus_disaster_center/resources/disaster_preparedness_for_pets.html. Accessed June 28, 2008.

25. The American Red Cross. Disaster services. Available at: http://www.redcross.org/services/disaster/0,0_500_,00.html,1081. Accessed June 28, 2008.

26. Homeland Security Presidential Directive–5. Available at: http://www.whitehouse.gov/news/releases/2003/02/print/20030228-9.html. Accessed June 28, 2008.

27. Introduction to ICS. In: EMI course number IS100 student manual 2005. Emmitsburg (MO): FEMA-Emergency Management Institute; 2005. p. 2–7, 4–4, 5–4.

28. Federal Emergency Management Agency. FEMA independent study program. Available at: http://training.fema.gov/IS/crslist.asp. Accessed July 25, 2008.

29. Emergency Management Institute. IS-701 NIMS multi agency coordination system course. Available at: http://training.fema.gov/EMIWeb/IS/is701.asp. Accessed June 28, 2008.

30. US Department of Health and Human Services. National Veterinary Response Team. Available at: http://www.hhs.gov/aspr/opeo/ndms/teams/vmat.html. Accessed June 28, 2008.

31. Gaylon J. A veterinarian's role in an animal health emergency . Emerging and exotic diseases of animals. Ames (IA): Iowa State University Institute for International Cooperation in Animal Biologics; 2006. p. 45, 52.

32. Animal Plant Health Inspection Service. Protect our animals. Protect our communities. [brochure]. Available at: http://www.aphis.usda.gov/publications/animal_health/content/printable_version/NAHERC-brochure-Vet-2007.pdf. Accessed June 28, 2008.

33. The Humane Society of the United States. How can I help. Available at: http://www.ndart.org/how/index.php. Accessed June 28, 2008.

34. United Animal Nations. Emergency animal rescue services. Available at: http://www.uan.org/index.cfm?navid=27. Accessed July 25, 2008.

35. American Humane Society. Red star animal emergency services. Available at: http://www.americanhumane.org/site/PageServer?pagename=pa_disaster_relief. Accessed July 25, 2008.

36. Federal Emergency Management Agency. Policy reference manual. Available at: http://fema.gov/pdf/government/grant/pa/policy.pdf. Accessed June 28, 2008.

37. Emergency Management Institute. Animals in disaster, module A. Awareness and preparedness. Available at: http://www.training.fema.gov/EMIWeb/IS/is10.asp. Accessed July 25, 2008.

Border Health: Who's Guarding the Gate?

Karen Ehnert, DVM, MPVM[a,b,]*, G. Gale Galland, DVM, MS[c]

KEYWORDS

- Importation • Trade • Animals • Zoonoses • Disease risk

IMPORTATION OF DOMESTIC AND EXOTIC PETS: CHANGES IN MARKET FORCES

The global trade market, the ease of transporting animals across continents and around the world, lower production costs in foreign countries, and market demand have resulted in a thriving pet trade of exotic animals, birds, and puppies, both pure-bred and small mixed breeds. The flood of animals crossing the United States' borders satisfies the public demand for these pets but is not without risk.

Trade barriers have been disappearing, creating a global marketplace. Improved transportation networks allow travelers, trade goods, and animals to move across continents or the globe in a single day. Improved communication and expanded use of the Internet for commerce simplify the connection between consumers and suppliers worldwide. These changes have created an environment in which a new global pet trade thrives.[1]

Between 1986 and 1993, the Uruguay Round of the General Agreement on Tariffs and Trade was held. The trade negotiations led to the creation of the World Trade Organization (WTO) in 1994 and the reduction of tariffs, import limits, and quotas over the next 20 years.[2] Agricultural product trade was liberalized, and guidelines on the trade of animals and animal products were created by the Office International des Epizooties.[3] The WTO operates under the principle that imported products be treated as favorably as domestic goods, but countries are permitted to take measures to protect humans and animals. These changes in trade regulations seem to have expanded the global market. The volume of world trade increased threefold from 1985 through 2000, and the export value of goods from Asia increased fivefold.[4]

Exotic pet ownership is on the rise in the United States, resulting in an increased trade in live animals. The number of United States households owning reptiles

The findings and conclusions in the manuscript are those of the authors and do not necessarily represent the views of the Centers for Disease Control and Prevention.
[a] Los Angeles County Department of Public Health, Veterinary Public Health & Rabies Control, 7601 E. Imperial Highway, Building 700, Suite 94A, Downey, CA 90242, USA
[b] College of Veterinary Medicine, Western University of Health Sciences, Pomona, CA, USA
[c] United States Public Health Services, Centers for Disease Control and Prevention, Division of Global Migration and Quarantine, 1600 Clifton Road, M/S E03, Atlanta, GA 30333, USA
* Corresponding author.
E-mail address: kehnert@ph.lacounty.gov (K. Ehnert).

Vet Clin Small Anim 39 (2009) 359–372
doi:10.1016/j.cvsm.2008.10.012
0195-5616/08/$ – see front matter © 2009 Elsevier Inc. All rights reserved.
vetsmall.theclinics.com

increased from 850,000 in 1991 to 2.7 million in 1998, and from 2001 to 2006 the numbers of pet birds, rodents, fish, turtles, and lizards have risen.[5] Importers, both legal and illegal, have stepped forward to meet this demand. In the early 1990s, United States imports and exports accounted for 80% of the total world trade of approximately 70 reptile species listed under the Convention on International Trade in Endangered Species of Wild Fauna and Flora (CITES).[6] In the United States, the annual volume of live animal imports has roughly doubled since 1991.[1] There were 183,000 wildlife shipments in 2006, with a declared value of more than $2.1 billion.[7] From 2003 through 2006, annual increases in wildlife trade ranged from 6% to 11%. From 2000 through 2004, approximately 588,000 animals were imported into the United States each day.[1]

The number of animals being imported illegally is difficult to estimate. Wildlife smuggling is very profitable and is estimated to bring in more than $6 billion each year.[8] Interpol estimates that wildlife smuggling ranks third on the contraband list of items of value, behind drugs and firearms.[8] Customs officers have found animals stuffed in clothing, bags, containers, compartments in cars, and even inside artificial limbs. Animal smuggling is likely to continue until the penalties outweigh the profits.

Starting in 2001, the Los Angeles County Veterinary Public Health and Rabies Control program (VPH-RCP) noticed a sharp increase in puppies being imported from overseas, with an accompanying increase in public interest regarding how to import puppies for resale. Individuals have reported that imported puppies could be sold for much more than their purchase price and shipment costs (VPH-RCP, unpublished data). A kennel in Los Angeles County is selling Yorkshire terrier puppies imported from South Korea for $1500 to $4000 each. Puppies smuggled from Mexico often are sold for $300 to $1000 cash. Small purebred or crossbred puppies are very popular,[9] and there is a lack of local breeders to meet the demand. The public's demand for small, cute puppies continues to stimulate the business and increase profits to puppy importers.

CHALLENGES WITH OVERSIGHT AND REGULATION OF TRADE: WHO'S IN CHARGE?

Requirements for importing animals into the United States can be found in the regulations of several federal agencies and reflect the mission of each agency.

In 1900, the Lacey Act became the first federal law protecting wildlife, by prohibiting the interstate movement and importation of wildlife species.[10] Additionally, the Lacey Act prohibits the importation of wildlife that has been determined to be injurious to people, agriculture, horticulture, forestry, or wildlife in the United States[1] In 1940, the Bureau of Fisheries and the Bureau of Biological Survey was consolidated to create the United States Fish and Wildlife Service (USFWS) in the Department of the Interior,[11] with the mission of conserving and protecting wildlife and plants. In 1973, the Endangered Species Act was passed to protect endangered or threatened species.[10] The USFWS also enforces requirements for CITES, an international agreement between governments to ensure that international trade in wild animals and plants does not threaten the existence of those species.[12] Lists of endangered or threatened species covered under CITES can be found in Appendices I, II, and III of the agreement.[13]

USFWS regulations require that all wildlife species imported for commercial, noncommercial, scientific, or personal use be declared at the time of import, be cleared by the USFWS, and enter the United States through a designated port. In most cases, the importer must have a USFWS permit.[14,15] If the species is covered under CITES, the shipment also must be accompanied by a current CITES certificate.[12]

The US Department of Agriculture (USDA) Animal and Plant Health Inspection Service (APHIS)[16] was established in 1972 to protect United States agriculture, consolidating the functions of previous animal and plant bureaus within the USDA. The basis for APHIS came from the USDA's first regulatory program, the Veterinary Division, established in 1883. In 1884, the Veterinary Division became the Bureau of Animal Industry, which was created by Congress to promote research in livestock diseases, enforce animal import regulations, and regulate the interstate movement of animals. In 1953, the USDA's Agriculture Research Service replaced the Bureau of Animal Industry. In 1971, the Agriculture Research Service became the Animal and Plant Health Service (APHS), and in 1972 the meat and poultry inspection divisions of the Consumer and Marketing Service were added, changing APHS to APHIS. Since 1972, several changes have occurred, including the establishment of the Food Safety and Quality Service, known today as USDA's Food Safety and Inspection Service, the transfer of the animal quarantine inspection activities at ports of entry from the Veterinary Services division to the Plant Protection division in 1974, and the movement of the port inspection activities to the Department of Homeland Security in 2002.[16–18]

USDA, APHIS Veterinary Services limits the importations of animals, animal products, and plants based on the risk to agriculture. Examples of these activities are controlling the importation of hoofed stock from countries in which foot and mouth disease is endemic or birds from countries that are experiencing outbreaks of highly pathogenic avian influenza (H5N1) in poultry. Importation of livestock or other hoofed stock, birds, dogs, or other animals may require a permit and possibly quarantine in a USDA facility before the shipment is allowed to enter the United States.[19]

The Animal Welfare Act was passed in 1966 to require minimum standards of animal care for animals that are used in research, bred for sale or exhibition, or transported commercially. APHIS' Animal Care program enforces the provisions of the Animal Welfare Act and the Horse Protection Act, which was passed by Congress in 1970.[20] The Animal Care program ensures that all animals are transported at the proper ages, in proper crates, and in appropriate conditions in accordance with the Animal Welfare Act. The Animal Care program does not have regulations specific to importation of animals.

The Centers for Disease Control and Prevention (CDC) of the Department of Health and Human Services has regulations prohibiting or controlling the importation of a variety of species of animals and animal products based on a specific threat to human health. For example, dogs entering the United States from countries reporting cases of rabies need proof of a current rabies vaccination, or the importer must sign an agreement to confine the animal until appropriate vaccinations can be obtained and then for an additional 30 days after vaccination. The importation of nonhuman primates has been regulated since 1975, limiting their importation specifically to purposes of science, education, or exhibition and requiring that importers be registered by the CDC. In 2003, importation of civets was banned because these animals were considered to be an amplifying host or vector for severe acute respiratory syndrome (SARS). In 2003, the importation of African rodents was banned in response to an outbreak of monkeypox in the United States associated with imported Gambian pouched rats.[21]

Customs and Border Protection (CBP), located in the Department of Homeland Security, is the first line of defense at the border to ensure that animals and animal products are being imported in accordance with all federal agency regulations. Additionally, CBP has the authority to levy a fee on imported animals or products for commercial use, in accordance with the tariff codes.[22]

Animal importation regulations change often, reflecting any new disease threats that arise, and imported animals may require permits or approvals from a variety of agencies. Individuals planning to import animals should check with the USDA, CDC, USFWS, and CPB to make certain that all required documents are obtained before an animal is brought to the United States.

BORDER PUPPIES: A GROWING PROBLEM

In California, the number of legally documented dog imports began increasing in 2001 (**Fig. 1**). In 2000, most imported dogs were single imports. Some were personal pets; others were purebred dogs that had been purchased from an overseas breeder. Few dogs were imported for resale. In 2003, the number of imports of multiple puppies per shipment began to increase. The number of puppies imported into California through airports has increased from 110 multidog imports documented in 2003 to 365 in 2004 and 341 in 2005. Each shipment contained as many as 40 puppies. Such large numbers of puppies are being imported for resale and not as personal pets. A similar increase was seen nationally.[23] An estimated 287,000 dogs were imported into the United States in 2006, with 70,600 lacking proof of valid rabies vaccinations, mostly because they were too young to be vaccinated.[23] In California, most of the imported puppies were destined for Los Angeles County (**Fig. 2**), and the most common countries of origin were Mexico and Canada (**Fig. 3**). Many dogs also were imported from Asia, Europe, South America, and Russia. In Los Angeles County, many puppies were imported from South Korea by pet stores or kennels. The most common breed imported was Yorkshire terrier, followed by Maltese, bulldogs, and poodles (**Fig. 4**).

As the number of shipments containing more than one dog increased, tracking puppies became increasingly more difficult in Los Angeles County. Initially, several shipments went to local pet stores, but as Los Angeles County VPH-RCP staff began enforcing postimportation quarantines until 30 days after the puppies received their rabies immunization, shipments became harder to locate. Puppies were sold before

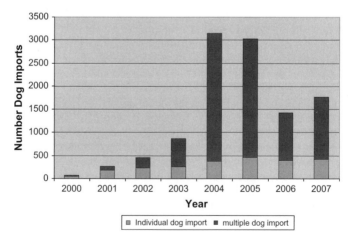

Fig. 1. Number of dogs imported individually or in a group into California, 2000 through 2007, for which CDC confinement was completed and submitted to the California Department of Public Health. The data do not include legally and illegally imported puppies that were not identified by CDC officers. (*Data from* California Department of Public Health, Veterinary Public Health Section, Sacramento, CA.)

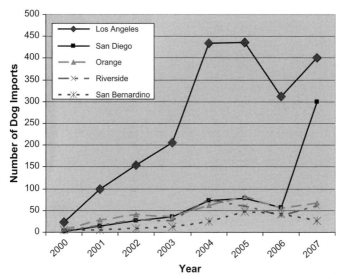

Fig. 2. Number of dogs imported into California, by top five counties and year (2000–2007) for which CDC confinement was completed and submitted to the California Department of Public Health. The data do not include legally and illegally imported puppies that were not identified by CDC officers. (*Data from* California Department of Public Health, Veterinary Public Health Section, Sacramento, CA.)

VPH-RCP visits, incorrect addresses were indicated on the CDC confinement agreement form, and individuals refused entrance onto their properties. In addition, some importers provided falsified rabies certificates, and puppies were not available for inspection. This problem was not limited to Los Angeles County. New York City

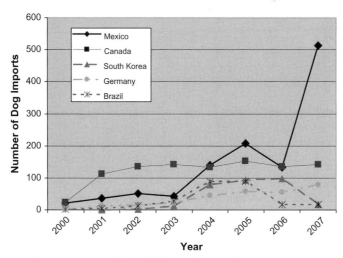

Fig. 3. Number of dogs imported into California by top five countries of origin and year (2000–2007) for which CDC confinement was completed and submitted to the California Department of Public Health. The data do not include legally and illegally imported puppies that were not identified by CDC officers. (*Data from* California Department of Public Health, Veterinary Public Health Section, Sacramento, CA.)

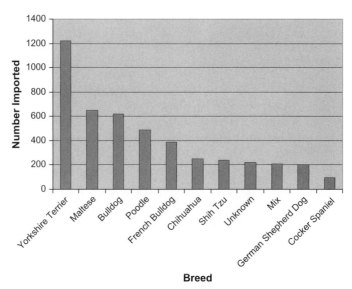

Fig. 4. Number of dogs imported into California by top 10 reported dog breeds, 2000 through 2007, for which CDC confinement was completed and submitted to the California Department of Public Health. The data do not include legally and illegally imported puppies that were not identified by CDC officers. (*Data from* California Department of Public Health, Veterinary Public Health Section, Sacramento, CA.)

sent out a veterinary alert in 2005 to notify veterinarians that puppies were being imported from rabies-endemic countries and that some were being sold without completing the mandated confinement.[24] The CDC noted more than 4000 confinement agreement violations among imported dogs in 2006.[23]

During the past few years, illegal shipments of puppies also have become a problem. The Los Angeles County VPH-RCP and animal law enforcement agencies throughout California began receiving reports in 2004 that individuals were purchasing puppies in Mexico and selling them in California. These puppies were advertised in free classified ads and were delivered to the purchaser at a public location, or they were sold directly from vehicles in shopping center parking lots. Generally, the purchaser was required to pay cash and had no way of contacting the seller after purchase. Many of the puppies were ill and died a short time after being sold to unsuspecting buyers (personal communication, Captain Aaron Reyes, Southeast Area Animal Control Authority, December 4, 2007).

In early 2005, 14 animal law enforcement agencies and three health agencies, including the Los Angeles County VPH-RCP, formed the Border Puppy Task Force (BPTF) to assess this growing and disturbing trend.[25] In December 2005, animal law enforcement officers worked alongside CBP agents for a 2-week period, examining and documenting animals entering from Mexico through two California border crossings. More than 500 puppies were examined during this operation; many were found huddled together in cardboard boxes in car trunks or wrapped in towels and stuffed under seats (**Fig. 5**).[25] Only a few puppies were confiscated because of illness. Most were allowed to enter California after a CDC confinement order was issued. These numbers indicate that 10,000 or more puppies may be imported each year through the two California–Mexico border crossings investigated, and few are confined as required by federal law to protect against introduction of rabies.

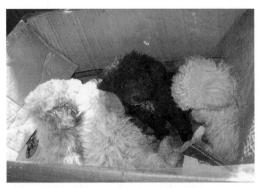

Fig. 5. Puppies discovered in a vehicle at one of two California–Mexico border crossings during a Border Puppy Task Force operation. (*Photograph courtesy of* Captain Aaron Reyes, Southeast Area Animal Control Authority, Downey, CA.)

Following the joint investigation, the BPTF held a news conference and conducted media interviews to educate the public about the risks associated with illegally imported puppies. Buyers were encouraged not to purchase puppies if the seller required cash and required that the puppy be delivered to its new owner in a public place, such as a restaurant or shopping center parking lot. Individuals whose puppy became ill or died shortly after purchase were encouraged to report the matter to the BPTF for follow-up investigation of illegal importers. In 2006 and 2007, the BPTF identified continued transport of puppies across the same border crossings. (personal communication, Captain Aaron Reyes, Southeast Area Animal Control Authority, December 4, 2007).

The CDC has responded to complaints about large-volume shipments of puppies intended for immediate resale and the need for additional regulations to prevent the introduction of zoonotic diseases into the United States by publishing an Advance Notice of Proposed Rulemaking on July 31, 2007.[26] Public comments were solicited until December 2007 and are being evaluated. Stakeholders were asked questions such as

Should the CDC establish a minimum age for importation of dogs, cats and ferrets?
Should imported animals have a unique identifier (microchip, tattoo)?
Should a valid international health certificate be required?
Should the importation of dogs, cats and ferrets be restricted to ports staffed by CDC quarantine personnel?

These changes could have a major impact on the legal and illegal international puppy trade. Until the regulations are revised, however, the flow of puppies into the United States is likely to continue.

ANIMAL SPECIES AND POTENTIAL DISEASE RISKS

The worldwide movement of animals increases the potential for the spread of diseases that pose a risk to human and animal health.[27,28] Animals are imported into the United States for use as pets, food and other animal products, scientific research, and exhibition in zoos. Dogs and cats are allowed to enter the country without health certificates and, if the owners sign a confinement agreement as described previously, without proof of rabies immunization. Even if a pet is ill on arrival, it may be allowed in, with a recommendation that the owner take the pet to a veterinarian for examination.[22] Many of the exotic animals are wild caught, and often there is no requirement that they be screened for zoonotic disease before or after arrival in the United States. Global trade of animals creates circumstances in which diseases that generally are not found in the United States may be introduced.

On the first World Rabies Day, September 8, 2007, the CDC reported that the canine strain of rabies had been eliminated from the United States The importation of dogs from rabies-enzootic countries represents a risk for reintroducing canine rabies.[27,29] Imported dogs have been found to be infected with rabies[24,27,30,31] on several occasions. In 1988, a 5-month-old puppy imported from Mexico into New Hampshire became ill 3 weeks after its arrival.[30] The dog began whimpering and had tremors in one leg for 3 days. It then developed urinary and fecal incontinence and finally excessive salivation. The owners took the puppy to a veterinarian, who suspected rabies based on the puppy's history and clinical signs. The puppy was euthanized, tested, and found to be rabid. Seventeen people had been exposed, including the owner's classmates, partygoers, and a babysitter. In 2004, a 3-month-old ill puppy was imported from Thailand through the Los Angeles International Airport and was allowed to enter the country.[31] It had been evaluated by several veterinarians in Thailand for a respiratory illness and had begun vomiting while in flight. The owner took the puppy to three veterinary clinics as she traveled to her home in Northern California. The puppy was aggressive and seemed to have pain along its back. Obvious neurologic signs did not develop until it was seen at the third veterinary clinic. At that point, the puppy was euthanized and tested positive for rabies (Thai canine variant). Numerous people had been exposed, and 12 individuals required postexposure prophylaxis.[27] More recently, in 2007, a puppy imported from India by a Washington State veterinarian developed rabies after being adopted by another veterinarian and taken to Alaska.[27] The puppy became ill 2 days after arrival from India, with at least one episode of regurgitation. It then bit one of the veterinarians and another dog. Clinic staff noticed it gnawing on its kennel, resulting in bleeding gums. Even so, another veterinarian completed a health certificate for the puppy, and a third veterinarian transported it to Alaska. The day after arriving in Alaska, the puppy developed neurologic signs and died. The puppy was tested and found to be rabid (Indian canine rabies variant); eight individuals received rabies postexposure prophylaxis.

Previous documented vaccination does not always negate the risk of imported rabies. In 1986, a dog developed rabies 10 months after being imported from Cameroon.[32] The dog had been vaccinated against rabies twice in West Africa and once after arriving in the United States The owners took the dog to an animal hospital after it developed paralysis of the lower jaw. The dog was docile and ambulatory. It was discharged with a diagnosis of "viral infection," and the owner was directed to force feed it. The dog was seen at two different clinics over 4 days and finally was euthanized and tested for rabies. It was found to have a West African dog strain of rabies. Thirty-seven individuals received postexposure prophylaxis after potential exposures to the dog during its illness and the 2 weeks before the onset of clinical signs.

In 1987, an ill cat from Mexico also was allowed to enter the country through Los Angeles International Airport.[30] The cat was seen by three veterinarians before being euthanized and testing positive for rabies.

Other countries have reported imported rabies cases. France has identified several cases of rabies in dogs imported illegally from Morocco through Portugal or Spain by car.[33–35] In 2004 and again in 2007, three cases of canine rabies were reported in imported dogs. In 2007, Belgium and Germany also reported rabies in dogs imported illegally from Morocco.[36,37]

Imported dogs may carry other diseases, such as screwworm,[38,39] that pose risk to both animals and humans. Screwworm infestation begins when a female fly lays eggs on a superficial wound. Unlike typical maggots that feed on dead tissue, the screwworm feeds on living tissue. One female fly may lay up to 400 eggs at a time and as many as 2800 eggs during a 31-day lifespan. The eggs hatch into larvae that burrow into the wound and begin feeding on living flesh. After feeding for 5 to 7 days, the larvae drop off and burrow into the soil, where they pupate. The adult screwworm fly emerges and then mates after 3 to 5 days.[40]

In the first day or two of screwworm infection, the clinical signs include a slight motion inside the wound and possibly a serosanguineous discharge and a distinctive odor. By the third day, the larvae may be seen easily. In dogs, the larvae often tunnel under the skin, and there may be a large pocket of larvae with only a small opening in the skin. The deep burrowing is distinctive of screwworms, because other types of maggots are surface feeders and feed on dead tissue. If screwworms are left untreated, animals may die of secondary infection or toxicity within 7 to 14 days of infection. Daily wound treatment and larvicidal insecticides are necessary to control the screwworm larvae.[40]

In 2007, astute veterinarians in Mississippi and Massachusetts identified screwworm larvae in imported dogs.[38,39] Both New World (*Cochliomyia hominovorax*) and Old World (*Chyrsoma bezziana*) screwworm myiasis are considered foreign animal diseases in the United States and are reportable within 24 hours of diagnosis. New World screwworms were eradicated from the United States in 1966. The Old World screwworm had never been seen in this country until it was found in a 1-year-old dog imported from Singapore to Massachusetts in October 2007. In September 2007, a 16-year-old dog was imported from Trinidad and entered the country through the Miami airport.[41] It was seen by a Mississippi veterinarian 3 days after arrival for ocular damage caused by larval infection. In both cases, the practitioners recognized that the larvae seemed unusual and submitted specimens for identification. Their quick action prevented these insects from becoming established, which could have resulted in the United States livestock industry suffering $750 million in production losses.[38]

Imported dogs may introduce other non-native pathogens to the United States. In 1991, a dog imported from England to Canada was found to be infected with *Angiostrongylus vasorum*, a nematode parasite of the pulmonary arteries and right heart of dogs and wild carnivores.[42] This parasite is enzootic among dogs in areas of Europe and Uganda but is not considered established in North America. In 2005, an investigation in French Guiana, South America, determined that a dog imported from France in 2002 had *Leishmania infantum* and subsequently spread the infection to a second dog.[43]

Imported wild or exotic animals also pose a risk to human and animal health. Bats have been associated with rabies virus and related lyssaviruses, Nipah and Hendra viruses, and a SARS-like virus of bats.[44] A highly pathogenic strain of the influenza virus, H5N1 (HPAI), first appeared in Asia in 1997 and subsequently spread to Russia, Europe, and parts of Africa.[45] Live bird markets, trade, wild birds, and illegal bird importation probably all contributed to the spread of the disease.[46,47] In 2004, two crested hawk-eagles that had been smuggled into Europe from Thailand were seized at the Brussels International Airport. Although neither appeared ill, they were euthanized and were found to be infected with HPAI.

Bird smuggling continues to be a problem in the United States. From 1999 through 2004, federal authorities intercepted 30 individuals attempting to smuggle commercial quantities of live birds into the United States from Mexico.[48] Before being arrested, one individual had illegally transported between 6000 and 10,000 exotic birds, valued at more than $1.5 million, across the border. Smuggled birds are not quarantined, screened, or treated as required by federal law. In addition to avian influenza, smuggled birds may carry exotic Newcastle disease, a foreign animal disease that is lethal to poultry,[49,50] or avian chlamydiosis, a zoonosis that people can contract through contact with pet birds.[51]

Rodents, rabbits, and pocket pets also may pose a risk to human and animal health. In May and June 2003, the first cluster of human monkeypox cases in the United States was reported.[52] Many of the patients developed a febrile vesicular rash after having contact with prairie dogs that had acquired the infection through contact with a shipment of African rodents at a wholesale pet store.[53] The prairie dogs exhibited anorexia, wasting, sneezing, coughing, swollen eyelids, and ocular discharge.[52] Ultimately, there were 47 confirmed and probable human cases of monkeypox during this outbreak.[54] The traceback investigation showed that rodents imported from Africa were held in the same area as prairie dogs before being shipped to other distributors and, ultimately, to many pet stores. The frequent mixing of species in the wildlife trade arena creates an opportunity for cross-species transmission and the introduction of new diseases to domesticated animals, wildlife, and humans.[1]

In addition to zoonotic threats, imported animals may pose a risk to agriculture. Rabbit hemorrhagic disease (RHD) first was identified in China in 1984. RHD is a highly contagious calicivirus that kills up to 90% of infected animals.[55] Infected rabbits often develop a blood-tinged foamy nasal discharge, severe respiratory distress, and/or convulsions before death. In 5% to 10% of the rabbits, clinical signs do not progress as rapidly but may include jaundice, malaise, weight loss, and eventually death in 1 to 2 weeks. This disease has spread to Europe, Asia, Australia, New Zealand, and Cuba but still is considered a foreign animal disease in the United States. Outbreaks of RHD occurred in the United States in 2000, 2001, and 2005.[56] The 2005 outbreak of RHD occurred at a rabbitry in Indiana after the owner purchased 11 rabbits from a flea market in Kentucky. Following the introduction of the new rabbits, nearly half of his herd died, and the remaining animals were euthanized to contain the outbreak. The source of the infection never was determined.

Imported exotic pets also may carry parasites that could pose a public health or agricultural health threat. In 1999, Florida animal health officials detected exotic ticks on a leopard tortoise that contained *Cowdria ruminantium*, the cause of heartwater disease in ruminants.[57]

SUMMARY

Imported dogs bring the risk of the reintroduction of canine rabies, screwworm, and other diseases. Exotic birds pose a risk for avian influenza, exotic Newcastle disease, and psittacosis. Rodents have been a source of imported monkeypox, and turtles can carry ticks that spread heartwater disease. Regulations are in place to reduce the risk of diseases that pose a threat to public health and agriculture from imported animals. Changes to the regulations are being proposed to define better the United States entry and follow-up requirements. Veterinarians play an essential role in preventing the transmission of zoonotic disease between animals and the public and are on the front line dealing with imported animals. They should be aware of and compliant with state and local regulations and play an active role in educating and advising clients regarding the risk of importing an animal. Veterinarians should be vigilant when examining new puppies. Many imported dogs never are confined properly or inspected for infectious diseases, and many diseases may not be detected readily in imported dogs. With the current rabies vaccination requirements in the United States, most veterinarians have never seen a pet with rabies and do not consider rabies in the differential diagnosis. Additionally, early signs of rabies may be very subtle and may not be recognized readily. It is important to keep rabies on the differential list, especially if the pet is known to have been or is suspected of having been imported. Additional training in recognizing emerging infectious diseases may be helpful. Veterinarians should contact their local health department immediately about any potential rabies cases or suspicious illness, especially in imported animals. A veterinarian could be the one who prevents the next outbreak.

ACKNOWLEDGEMENTS

The authors thank Dr. Ben Sun and Sharon Ernst who provided data on CDC confinement agreements completed for dogs imported into California.

REFERENCES

1. Jenkins PT, Genovese K, Ruffler H. Broken screens: the regulation of live animal importation in the United States. Washington, DC: Defenders of Wildlife; 2007. Available at: http://www.defenders.org/resources/publications/programs_and_policy/international_conservation/broken_screens/broken_screens_report.pdf. Accessed February 16, 2008.
2. Leslie J, Upton M. The economic implications of greater global trade in livestock and livestock products. Rev Sci Tech 1999;18(2):440–57.
3. Walton TE. The impact of diseases on the importation of animals and animal products. Ann N Y Acad Sci 2000;916:36–40.
4. Sutherst RW. Global change and human vulnerability to vector-borne diseases. Clin Microbiol Rev 2004;17(1):136–73.
5. Shepherd AJ. Results of the 2006 AVMA survey of companion animal ownership in US pet-owning households. J Am Vet Med Assoc 2008;232(5):695–6.
6. USDA/APHIS/VS, Centers for Epidemiology and Animal Health. The reptile and amphibian communities in the United States. Available at: http://www.aphis.usda.gov/vs/ceah/cei/bi/emergingmarketcondition_files/reptile.pdf. Accessed March 8, 2008.
7. US Fish and Wildlife Service, Office of Law Enforcement. Annual report FY 2006. Available at: http://www.fws.gov/le/pdffiles/AnnualReportFY2006.pdf; August 2007. Accessed March 8, 2008.
8. US Customs and Border Protection. All creatures great and small: wildlife smuggling "not worth the risk". US Customs Today January 2003. Available at: http://www.cbp.gov/xp/CustomsToday/2003/January/wildlife.xml. Accessed April 6, 2008.
9. American Kennel Club. AKC dog registration statistics. Available at: http://www.akc.org/reg/dogreg_stats.cfm. Accessed April 6, 2008.
10. U.S. Fish and Wildlife Service, Office of Law Enforcement. History. Available at: http://www.fws.gov/le/AboutLE/1900-1950.htm. Accessed April 18, 2008.
11. U.S. Fish and Wildlife Service. About the U.S. Fish and Wildlife Service. Available at: http://www.fws.gov/help/about_us.html. Accessed April 18, 2008.
12. Convention on International Trade in Endangered Species. Wild fauna and flora. Available at: http://www.cites.org/. Accessed April 18, 2008.
13. Convention on International Trade in Endangered Species. Wild fauna and flora. The CITES appendices. Available at: http://www.cites.org/eng/app/index.shtml. Accessed on April 18, 2008.

14. U.S. Fish and Wildlife Service. Import/export. Available at: http://www.fws.gov/le/ImpExp/Contact_Info_Ports.htm. Accessed April 18, 2008.
15. U.S. Fish and Wildlife Service, Office of Law Enforcement. Importing and exporting your commercial wildlife shipment. Available at: http://www.fws.gov/le/ImpExp/CommWildlifeImportExport.htm. Accessed April 18, 2008.
16. U.S. Department of Agriculture, Animal and Plant Health Inspection Service. About USDA, history of APHIS. Available at: http://www.aphis.usda.gov/about_aphis/history.shtml. Accessed April 18, 2008.
17. U.S. Department of Agriculture, Animal and Plant Health Inspection Service. Import export. Available at: http://www.aphis.usda.gov/import_export/index.shtml. November 8, 2007. Accessed April 18, 2008.
18. U.S. Department of Agriculture, Animal and Plant Health Inspection Service. Import export, animal and animal product import information, live animals. Available at: http://www.aphis.usda.gov/import_export/animals/live_animals.shtml. Accessed April 18, 2008.
19. U.S. Department of Agriculture, Animal and Plant Health Inspection Service. Animal health. Available at: http://www.aphis.usda.gov/animal_health/index.shtml. Accessed April 18, 2008.
20. U.S. Department of Agriculture, Animal and Plant Health Inspection Service. Animal welfare. Available at: http://www.aphis.usda.gov/animal_welfare/downloads/awa/54USC2131.txt. Accessed April 18, 2008.
21. Centers for Disease Control and PreventionDivision of Global Migration and Quarantine. Importation of pets, other animals, and animal products into the United States. Available at: http://www.cdc.gov/ncidod/dq/animal.htm. Accessed April 21, 2008.
22. U.S. Customs and Border Protection. Importing into the United States, a guide for commercial importers. Available at: http://www.cbp.gov/linkhandler/cgov/newsroom/publications/trade/iius.ctt/iius.doc. Accessed on April 21, 2008.
23. McQuiston JH, Wilson T, Harris S, et al. Importation of dogs into the United States: risks from rabies and other zoonotic diseases. Zoonoses Public Health. 02 Apr 2008. Published online. Available at: http://www.blackwell-synergy.com/doi/abs/10.1111/j.1863-2378.2008.01117.x. Accessed April 6, 2008.
24. City of New York, Department of Health and Mental Hygiene. 2005 Veterinary alert #1. Available at: http://www.nyc.gov/html/doh/downloads/pdf/zoo/05vet01.pdf. March 28, 2005;. Accessed March 8, 2008.
25. South East Area Animal Control Authority (SEAACA). Border Puppy Task Force … buyer beware. Available at: http://www.seaaca.org/BorderPuppyTaskForce.htm. Accessed April 6, 2008.
26. Centers for Disease Control and Prevention, HHS. Foreign quarantine regulations, proposed revision of HHS/CDC animal-import regulations. Fed Regist 2007;72(146):41676–9.
27. Castrodale L, Walker V, Baldwin J, et al. Rabies in a puppy imported from India to the USA, March 2007. Zoonoses Public Health. 7 Mar 2008. Published online. Available at: http://www.blackwell-synergy.com/doi/abs/10.1111/j.1863-2378.2008.01107.x?journalCode=jvb. Accessed April 18, 2008.
28. Marano N, Arguin PM, Pappaioanou M. Impact of globalization and animal trade on infectious disease ecology. Emerg Infect Dis 2007;13(12):1807–9.
29. CDC. Notice to readers: world rabies day. MMWR Morb Mortal Wkly Rep 2007; 56(35):915.
30. CDC. Epidemiologic notes and reports imported dogs and cat rabies—New Hampshire, California. MMWR Morb Mortal Wkly Rep 1988;37(36):559–60.

31. Santa Barbara County Public Health Department. Rabies in a puppy imported to California from Thailand. Epidemiology & Disease Control Newsletter. 2004;III(2):2. Available at: http://www.sbcphd.org/documents/dcp/newsletter_summer_2004.pdf. Accessed April 6, 2008.
32. CDC. An imported case of rabies in an immunized dog. MMWR Morb Mortal Wkly Rep 1987;36(7):94–6, 101.
33. Promed mail. Canine rabies in France. Promed mail 2008. Mar 7: 2080307.0938. Available at: http://www.promedmail.org. Accessed March 7, 2008.
34. Promed mail. Rabies, canine—France (02): investigation. Promed mail 2008. Mar 14: 20080314.1019. Available at: http://www.promedmail.org. Accessed March 14, 2008.
35. Servas V, Mailles A, Neau D, et al. An imported case of canine rabies in Aquitaine: investigation and management of the contacts at risk, August 2004–March 2005. Euro Surveill 2005;10(10–12):222–5.
36. Rabies News Archives. 29 October 2007. Belgium ex Morocco. Available at: http://www.rabies-vaccination.com/news-archive.asp. Accessed April 6, 2008.
37. Rabies New Archives. 20 April 2007. Germany, Hamburg ex Morocco. Available at: http://www.rabies-vaccination.com/news-archive.asp. Accessed April 6, 2008.
38. Wilson E, Eetherall K. Is it just another worble? California Veterinarian Jan–Feb 2008;62(1):14–5.
39. Scultz K. Dangerous screwworm species found in U.S., poses little threat. DVM Newsmagazine January 1, 2008. Available at: http://www.dvmnews.com/dvm/News/Dangerous-screwworm-species-found-in-US-poses-litt/ArticleStandard/Article/detail/485137. Accessed April 6, 2008.
40. The Center for Food Security & Public Health. Screwworm myiasis. October 3, 2007. Available at: http://www.cfsph.iastate.edu/FastFacts/pdfs/screwworm_myiasis_F.pdf. Accessed April 6, 2008
41. Smith D. Screwworm found in Mississippi dog. Available at: http://vetext.unl.edu/stories/200709250.shtml. Accessed April 23, 2008.
42. Perry AW, Herling R, Kennedy MJ. Angiostrongylosis with disseminated larval infection associated with signs of ocular and nervous disease in an imported dog. Can Vet J 1999;32:430–1.
43. Rotureau B, Ravel C, Aznar C, et al. First report of *Leishmania infantum* in French Guiana: canine visceral leishmaniasis imported from the old world. J Clin Microbiol 2006;44(3):1120–2.
44. Calisher CH, Childs JE, Field HE, et al. Bats: important reservoir hosts of emerging viruses. Clin Microbiol Rev 2006;19:531–45.
45. Alexander DJ. Summary of avian influenza activity in Europe, Asia, Africa and Australasia, 2002–2006. Avian Dis 2007;51(1 suppl):161–6.
46. Domenech J, Slingenbergh J, Martin V, et al. Disease intelligence for highly pathogenic avian influenza. Dev Biol (Basel) 2007;135:7–12.
47. Van Borm S, Thomas I, Hanquet G, et al. Highly pathogenic H5N1 Influenza virus in smuggled Thai eagles, Belgium. Emerg Infect Dis 2007;11(5):702–5.
48. U.S. Fish and Wildlife Service. Exotic parrots confiscated from smugglers returned to Mexico. Press release. August 22, 2007. Available at: http://www.fws.gov/news/NewsReleases/showNews.cfm?newsId=8ED7D2C7-0950-F2DB-9DB30E5A956367E5. Accessed April 20, 2008.
49. Bruning-Fann C, Kaneene J, Heamon J. Investigation of an outbreak of velogenic viscerotropic Newcastle disease in pet birds in Michigan, Indiana, Illinois and Texas. J Am Vet Med Assoc 1992;201(11):1709–14.

50. Seal BS, King DJ, Locke DP, et al. Phylogenetic relationships among highly virulent Newcastle disease virus isolates obtained from exotic birds and poultry from 1986 to 1996. J Clin Microbiol 1998;36(4):1141–5.
51. Moroney JF, Guevera R, Iverson C, et al. Detection of chlamydiosis in a shipment of pet birds, leading to recognition of an outbreak of clinically mild psittacosis in humans. Clin Infect Dis 1998;26(6):1425–9.
52. Guarner J, Johnson BJ, Paddock CD, et al. Monkeypox transmission and pathogenesis in Prairie dogs. Emerg Infect Dis 2004;10(3):426–31.
53. Reed KD, Melshi JW, Graham MB, et al. The detection of monkeypox in humans in the Western hemisphere. N Engl J Med 2004;350:342–50.
54. Reynolds MG, Davidson WB, Curns AT, et al. Spectrum of infection and risk factors for human monkeypox, United States, 2003. Emerg Infect Dis 2007;13(0): 1332–9.
55. McIntosh MT, Behen SC, Mohamed FM, et al. A pandemic strain of calicivirus threatens rabbit industries in the Americas. Virol J 2007;4:96.
56. Center for Emerging Issues, Veterinary Services, APHIS. Rabbit hemorrhagic disease, Indiana, June 15, 2005 Impact Worksheet. Available at: http://www.aphis.usda.gov/vs/ceah/cei/taf/iw_2005_files/domestic/rhd_indiana_061505_files/rhd_indiana_061505.htm. Accessed Jan 2, 2008.
57. Burrige MJ, Simmons LA, Simbi BH, et al. Evidence of Cowdria ruminantium infection (heartwater) in Amblyomma sparsum ticks found on tortoises imported into Florida. J Parasitol 2000;86(5):1135–6.

Local Veterinary Diagnostic Laboratory, a Model for the One Health Initiative

Gundula Dunne, DVM, MPVM*, Nikos Gurfield, DVM

KEYWORDS

• Veterinary public health • Public health • Epidemiology
• Animal health • Animal diagnostic laboratory • One health

The role of veterinary diagnostic laboratories (VDLs) in public health often is viewed as limited to agriculture and food safety. This narrow focus does not capitalize fully on their potential to impact public health. VDLs are run by states, universities, or private companies and range in their missions, but they generally are highly focused on animal health concerns, from companion animal diagnostics to monitoring for foreign animal diseases in livestock. Funding is a major determinant of the scope of a laboratory's activities. VDL funding is derived from a variety of private and public sources including departments of agriculture, universities, grants, and fees from animal owners. In comparison, funds for public health laboratories originate from public sources such as local, state, and federal budgets. The existence of two separate diagnostic systems for human and animal diseases poses some challenges, because VDL resources also are used to protect public health. For the One Health Initiative to succeed in "improving the lives of all species, both human and animal by the integration of medicine and veterinary medicine," the barriers between veterinary and public health laboratories must be surmounted so that limited resources can be maximized to benefit society as a whole.[1]

In San Diego County, the Office of the County Veterinarian (OCV) and the San Diego County Animal Disease Diagnostic Laboratory (ADDL) have taken steps to enhance communication and promote resource sharing across the fields of public health, animal health, agriculture, and environmental health. The mission of the OCV and the ADDL is to protect and improve the well being of animals, agriculture, people, and the environment through excellence in diagnostics, outreach, and education. This article highlights how the OCV and ADDL have served private veterinary practitioners and illustrates their successes and challenges in achieving their mission.

County of San Diego, Department of Agriculture, Weights, and Measures, Office of the County Veterinarian, Animal Disease Diagnostic Laboratory, 5555 Overland Avenue, Suite 4103, San Diego, CA 92123, USA
* Corresponding author.
E-mail address: gdunne@sdcounty.ca.gov (G. Dunne).

Vet Clin Small Anim 39 (2009) 373–384
doi:10.1016/j.cvsm.2008.10.018
0195-5616/08/$ – see front matter. Published by Elsevier Inc.

The OCV traces its origins back to the early twentieth century with the creation of the San Diego County Charter. The history of the OCV over the last 80 years provides a basis for understanding its diverse and complex roles in local government and public health. The County Veterinarian initially was a charter officer, called the "County Live-stock Inspector," who reported to the director of the California Department of Food and Agriculture (CDFA). In 1946, San Diego County assumed control of the CDFA's Livestock and Poultry Laboratory in San Diego and merged it with the Meat and Dairy Division of the County Health Department to form the County Livestock Department. This new department was directed by the County Livestock Inspector. In 1966, the title of County Livestock Inspector was changed to County Veterinarian, and the OCV was established to replace the County Livestock Department. Local county ordinances gave the OCV authority to "operate the County Veterinary Diagnostics Laboratory to diagnose diseases hazardous to animals or transmissible to man, including rabies, and maintain liaison with groups interested in livestock, health, sanitation, disease control, and enforcement."[2] In 1979, the OCV was returned to the San Diego County Department of Health Services. Budget pressures in 1993 resulted in the office being transferred to its present location in the San Diego County Department of Agriculture (**Fig. 1**).

Under the Office of the County Veterinarian, the original Livestock and Poultry Laboratory has evolved into the ADDL, which analyzes a broad spectrum of animals, ranging from fish to zebras, to protect animal and human health. Today the OCV includes the ADDL, a plant pathology laboratory, and an entomology program.

San Diego County covers 4200 square miles and is the third most populous county in California, with more than 3 million residents.[3] The ADDL has more than 16,000 clients and handles more than 3300 specimens each year. Its clients include the University of California, the US Navy, the Salk Institute, the Scripps Research Institute, the San Diego Zoologic Society, the US Department of Agriculture (USDA), other San Diego County departments (eg, the Public Health Service [PHS], the Public Health

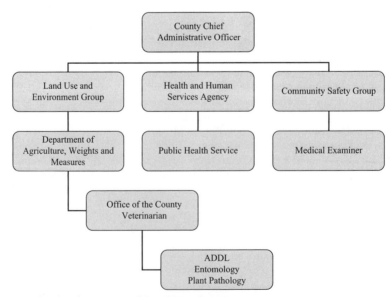

Fig. 1. Organizational structure of San Diego County.

Laboratory [PHL], and the Department of Animal Services), biotechnology companies, humane societies, Mexican health authorities at the Institute of Public Health Services of Baja California, wildlife rehabilitation groups, private veterinarians, farmers, and pet owners. For a nominal fee, the laboratory provides a wide range of diagnostic services: necropsies, microbiologic cultures, parasitology testing, serology, rabies testing, polymerase chain reaction (PCR) and electron microscopy, and microscopic examinations. The ADDL's work has been instrumental in preventing cases of human rabies, in convicting criminals of animal cruelty, in discovering new diseases, and in preventing entry of foreign animal diseases.

The ADDL's staff provides training to several groups, such as the USDA Wildlife Services, registered veterinary technicians, animal control personnel, and vocational programs. Additionally, the ADDL has created an internship program with educational opportunities for students, veterinarians, scholars, and pathologists from all over the world. The laboratory is a West Coast study site for the C.L. Davis Foundation for the Advancement of Veterinary and Comparative Pathology. This foundation's library has a collection of veterinary pathology resources including audio visual images and histopathology slides. The ADDL continually evaluates and disperses information about the status of communicable diseases in San Diego County to local health care providers and the community with quarterly publications, speaking engagements, weekly meetings with the PHS, and continuing education seminars.

BENEFITS OF A LOCAL VETERINARY DIAGNOSTIC LABORATORY

The ADDL provides its clients with diagnostic services in a timely and efficient manner. Rapid diagnostic results, coupled with direct communication between laboratory staff, local resource managers, and clients, enable appropriate, comprehensive local responses to be mounted against disease threats and other health concerns. This service has proved advantageous to the community in many instances. The convenient location of the ADDL facilitates sample submission and results in more submissions from a wide range of clients who normally would not submit samples to the nearest state VDL (the California Animal Health and Food Safety Laboratory, which is approximately 100 miles away). Moreover, unlike the state VDL, which does not accept companion animals such as dogs and cats, the ADDL accepts all animal species.

For necropsy, the ADDL encourages the submission of the complete body to allow the full range of diagnostic testing. Submission of the full body is preferable to piece-meal submission ("necropsy in a jar"). Such partial submissions typically fail to include all lesions and abnormal tissues and often preclude additional diagnostic testing such as bacterial culture, virus isolation, or toxicology. Also, improperly collected submissions can have artifacts from incomplete fixation or incorrect preservation. The local laboratory can be more accurate in disease assessment, especially in necropsies, because less information is lost through sample decomposition during shipping and handling. Furthermore, sending samples through a local VDL promotes the efficient use of resources, because specimens can be screened before reference laboratory resources are used for confirmatory testing.

The ADDL works with a diverse group of community partners and all levels of government. On a regular basis, the ADDL works with governmental agencies in public health, environmental health, agriculture, hazardous materials, water resources, parks and recreation, animal control, the military, and law enforcement. In the private sector, the ADDL serves wildlife rehabilitation groups, humane societies, farmers, veterinarians, bird stores, bird clubs, and private citizens. These relationships allow the ADDL to serve as a nexus among these groups to facilitate solutions to health threats. This nexus became especially apparent during preparations for highly pathogenic avian influenza H5N1, in which the OCV and the ADDL were the lead organizations for the county's avian influenza preparedness plan. The plan incorporates public and private resources to detect, contain, control, and recover from H5N1 or other novel avian influenza strains. Being locally based has allowed the ADDL to interpret and apply diagnostic information in the context of the local ecology and political dynamics, to achieve solutions that will be supported by the community and local government.

AVIAN DISEASE SURVEILLANCE

The original Livestock and Poultry Laboratory was established during the early twentieth century with the support of the large turkey industry in San Diego County. Diagnoses such as turkey pox, pullorum, and paratyphoid were common. Economic and urbanization pressures gradually reduced the poultry industry, but more than 2 dozen egg-laying and specialty poultry meat–producing farms with 1.5 million birds and $38 million in revenue still contribute to the county's agricultural industry.[4] The decrease in poultry operations has been counterbalanced by a growing exotic pet bird industry and by increased interest in diseases affecting wild bird populations.

Because of the economic ramifications of exotic Newcastle disease or H5N1 on domestic poultry operations, the avian disease surveillance program tests all birds submitted to the laboratory for these diseases, regardless of primary complaint. This policy has been in place for more than 50 years. Furthermore, San Diego's proximity to Mexico puts the county at risk for the importation of foreign animal diseases from Central and South America and Mexico. For example, H5N2 avian influenza, related to a Mexican lineage, was diagnosed in an Amazon parrot that was purchased from a San Diego street vendor in 2004 and, presumably, had been imported illegally from Mexico.[5] Thousands of birds enter the United States legally each year through the USDA Quarantine Station located on the southeastern border of the county with Mexico.[6] The Department of Homeland Security and the USDA intercept 500 to 1000 illegally imported birds each year; undoubtedly, many more enter unchecked.[7] Not only is San Diego at high risk for the introduction of novel avian influenza viruses via illegally smuggled birds, but the county is a major destination for migratory birds on the Pacific Flyway.

More than 490 different bird species are found in San Diego County, making it the most diverse bird population in any United States county.[8] The current US Interagency Strategic Plan for avian influenza surveillance focuses on the Alaskan flyway.[9] Many priority bird species in this plan, such as the northern pintail, mallard, black brant, red-throated loon and semipalmated plover, migrate through San Diego County.[9] An analysis by Kilpatrick and colleagues,[10] however, concluded that the entry of highly pathogenic avian influenza into the United States is most likely occur via migration of infected birds from South American countries rather than from Eastern Siberia. The analysis also concluded, "current American surveillance plans that focus primarily on the Alaskan migratory bird pathway may fail to detect the introduction of H5N1 into the US in time to prevent its spread into domestic poultry." The current focus on Alaska may miss infected transpacific long-range pelagic birds, the introduction of highly pathogenic strains resulting from mutations in low-pathogenic avian influenza viruses endemic to South America (ie, H7N3 in Bolivia and H5N2 in Mexico), or the introduction of highly pathogenic viruses into South America from other global regions.

The ADDL works with numerous partners, including the San Diego County Department of Environmental Health (DEH), the USDA, the US Fish and Wildlife Service, the US Navy, SeaWorld, Project Wildlife, parks departments, water authorities, lifeguards, and private citizens, to conduct surveillance for avian diseases important to public health and agriculture. These diseases include West Nile virus (WNV), avian influenza, exotic Newcastle disease, psittacosis, and salmonellosis. In 2007, more than 500 birds were submitted and tested for these diseases. This powerful community network provides the basis for ongoing avian disease surveillance, improving the likelihood of early detection and response to disease threats.

VECTOR-BORNE DISEASE SURVEILLANCE

A comprehensive vector-borne disease control program must include human, animal, and vector population surveillance. The ADDL and the DEH have collaborated to pool their resources and expertise efficiently to protect the county from vector-borne pathogens. San Diego County adopted the powers of a vector control district in 1989 for vector-borne disease surveillance and control to protect animals and people. Lacking a laboratory and the ability for in-house testing, the DEH program initially relied on out-of-county laboratories. Recognizing the benefits of local testing and surveillance of animals affected by vector-borne diseases, the DEH contracted with the ADDL to perform vector-borne disease testing in 1990.

Originally focused on Lyme disease and tularemia, the program expanded in 2006 into a comprehensive WNV dead-bird surveillance program, in which dead corvids and other selected bird species were retrieved by DEH staff for testing at the ADDL. The emergence of H5N1 presented an additional disease risk to wild bird populations. To minimize the chance of missing H5N1 infection in birds, the WNV dead-bird surveillance program was expanded to include avian influenza testing. The WNV dead-bird surveillance program quickly evolved into the current Dead Bird Reporting Hotline for response to WNV, H5N1, or other zoonotic diseases affecting birds. The dead-bird surveillance program has led to other discoveries, for example, the finding of a *Chlamydophila* epizootic in raptors during late 2007 (Nikos Gurfield, DVM, unpublished data, 2008). The collaboration between the ADDL and the DEH has yielded more rapid and accurate detection of WNV than either program could have attained alone. For example, the first indication of WNV activity in San Diego County, in 2003, was from birds submitted directly to the ADDL for necropsy, rather than through the DEH Dead Bird Reporting Hotline. From January to July 2008, the DEH has submitted 305 birds to the ADDL for testing through the Dead Bird Reporting Hotline, of which 36% tested positive for WNV.

The detection of the WNV-infected birds enables a proactive response that reduces the threat to animals and people. For instance, vector control teams from the DEH are sent to the areas where WNV-positive birds were collected to treat or eliminate any mosquito breeding sources. Press releases are used to disseminate information about disease transmission and prevention measures, such as methods for reducing mosquito exposure and eliminating stagnant water sources. Although WNV exhibits a seasonal pattern, testing and monitoring is performed year-round in San Diego County because of its mild climate that is conducive to year-round mosquito presence. Analyzing year-round trends is necessary for the application of optimal mosquito-control measures.

Tularemia is another disease that has been addressed effectively through collaboration between the ADDL and the DEH. In 2004, a concerned citizen reported a die-off of wild rabbits near a golf course in the northern part of the county. ADDL pathologists performed complete necropsies on several rabbits that had gross and histologic lesions consistent with tularemia. Cultures from affected tissues confirmed the presence of *Francisella tularensis*. In response, the DEH Vector Control initiated increased tick surveillance throughout the county to determine the geographic risk. Ticks from other regions of the county tested positive by PCR. Unexpectedly, many positive ticks were determined to be infected with a novel *Francisella*-like endosymbiont organism.[11] The potential pathogenicity of the endosymbiont is unknown at this time.

The ADDL and the DEH continue to test ticks for tularemia and other tick-borne pathogens. In 2007, the DEH submitted 183 tick pools (average 10 ticks per pool) to the ADDL for routine tularemia surveillance and submitted 40 pools for Lyme disease testing. In San Diego County, the prevalence of *F. tularensis* and *Borrelia burgdorferi* in ticks is low. Tick-borne disease surveillance presents an opportunity for rapid response to prevent the spread of these diseases if a positive sample is detected. The partnership of pathologists, epidemiologists, molecular biologists, vector ecologists, and entomologists in vector-borne disease surveillance helps to protect the county more effectively from these endemic and emerging vector-borne diseases.

SURVEILLANCE FOR *CHLAMYDOPHILIA PSITTACI*

Although the California Department of Public Health requires reporting of psittacosis in humans, and the CDFA requires reporting of avian chlamydiosis in poultry, no California laws require reporting of psittacosis in pet birds.[12,13] This omission leaves a large segment of the bird and human population vulnerable to *Chlamydophilia psittaci* infection. The ADDL attempts to mitigate this risk by working with community partners such as private veterinarians, the state VDL, the PHS, and the DEH to encourage voluntary reporting of both suspected and confirmed cases in human and birds. The ADDL investigates psittacosis reports from any source. Both the DEH and the PHS are notified of the reports, and these agencies actively co-investigate when pet stores or human cases are involved, respectively. The County Veterinarian places a quarantine order on positive-testing birds and on any exposed birds for 45 days, during which time the birds must complete appropriate treatment as prescribed by the owner's private veterinarian. Although pet bird cases are not reportable, the cases are reported voluntarily to the California Department of Public Health.

The ADDL has tested birds for avian chlamydiosis since the 1960s. Unfortunately, reporting and testing of birds decreased dramatically after 1997, when the California State legislature repealed the requirement for banding of budgies,[14] eliminating a means of regulating this population. The ADDL recorded a total 268 birds with avian chlamydiosis (51 confirmed cases) from 1989 to 1997. In contrast, from 1998 to 2007, there were only 84 recorded cases of avian chlamydiosis. At this time, the ADDL tests all necropsied birds for *Chlamydophila psittaci*. Among 1608 necropsied birds tested between 1998 and 2007, 31 were positive for *C. psittaci*. During this same period, the PHS reported one confirmed human case.[14]

A 2006 psittacosis investigation illustrates the direct impact of VDLs on public health. The ADDL was contacted by the PHS regarding a 50-year-old woman who had a suspected diagnosis of psittacosis. The woman's history included the death of a pet bird purchased 3 weeks before the onset of her symptoms. The woman's serologic titers for psittacosis were negative, possibly because of early intervention with azithromycin.[15] The patient's clinical signs and the diagnosis of pleuritis by MRI were consistent with psittacosis. The dead bird, necropsied by the ADDL, had gross and microscopic lesions, highly suggestive of *C. psittaci* infection. PCR testing confirmed the diagnosis. To prevent further cases, the bird store was quarantined for 45 days, all exposed birds were treated, and bird sales were halted during the first 7 days of the quarantine period. No further human or bird cases were found or reported. This investigation was a collaborative effort between the OCV, the ADDL, the DEH, the PHS, the bird's veterinarian, and the patient's physician. By partnering with other government agencies and promoting voluntary disease reporting, the OCV continues to mitigate the risk of psittacosis.

RABIES TESTING

Understanding that the rabies transmission cycle inextricably links human and animal health is the cornerstone of the collaboration and diagnostic partnership between the ADDL and the San Diego County PHL for rabies control and prevention. Rabies testing in San Diego County began in 1922 when dog rabies was endemic. Continuous yearly outbreaks in dogs occurred until 1954, finally tapering off with the implementation of rabies control programs that included licensing and vaccination requirements.[16,17] In San Diego County, the last dog rabies case occurred in 1969. The first case of bat rabies in San Diego County was diagnosed in 1963. The rabies diagnostic testing partnership between the PHL and the ADDL maximizes rabies surveillance by testing suspected-rabid animals with and without human exposure. Without this collaboration, more than 80% of the positive rabies cases would have gone undetected, and all the rabies cases in nonendemic species would have been missed.[18]

Most animals are submitted from animal control agencies, but any county resident including veterinarians, rescue organizations, zoos, and pet stores can submit an animal for rabies testing. Between 1979 and 2002, both the ADDL and the PHL performed rabies testing for the adjacent city of Tijuana, Mexico. The ADDL and the PHL tested a total of 13,189 animals from San Diego County (11,925) and Tijuana (1264) for rabies between January 1, 1995 and December 31, 2006. Seventy-two percent of the San Diego–origin animals involved human bite or other exposure; 22% had no human exposure reported; human exposure was unknown for 6%. Eighty-five percent of the animals submitted from Mexico had no reported human exposure; the remaining 15% involved human exposure.

The ADDL detected three cases of rabies in terrestrial wildlife from 1995 through July 2008. In 1997, a skunk from northern San Diego County was submitted by an animal control agency. The skunk had been acting abnormally near a house. The initial rabies test results by ADDL were indeterminate; subsequent testing by the Centers for Disease Control and Prevention (CDC) confirmed the skunk as positive with a bat strain of rabies. In 2000, a gray fox bitten by a dog was submitted by the California Department of Fish and Game and tested positive for a bat strain of rabies. In 2005, a skunk submitted by an animal control agency from central San Diego County was positive for a bat strain of rabies. No human exposures were reported in any of these cases.

The large volume of rabies tests performed in San Diego result in part from the accessibility of the ADDL, the recognition of the staff expertise, and the policy of free testing for any suspected-rabid animals, without regard to human exposure. This approach yields a more comprehensive assessment of the status of rabies in nonendemic species and can aid in the identification of unrecognized human rabies exposures, especially for bats, because people are more likely to recall a potential non-bite exposure during further questioning. Early recognition of a novel rabies strain can play a critical role in preventing its spread, introduction, or establishment. The majority of rabies testing in high-risk wild animals was performed at the ADDL. If this testing were stopped, there would be a substantial deficit in the rabies surveillance of wild mammals in San Diego County.

ANIMAL ABUSE CASES

Research indicates that animal abuse is linked to violence directed at humans, such as domestic violence and child abuse.[19] The ADDL performs necropsy examinations for animal abuse cases. Cases are submitted regularly by animal control, humane societies, the sheriff and police departments, and the district attorney. Necropsy reports that describe lesions consistent with witness accounts or that have evidence of animal abuse are used to prosecute suspects. Prosecutors have stated that suspects are more willing to take a plea bargain when faced with the weight of the evidence from a supportive necropsy report, thus saving the prosecution considerable time and money. ADDL pathologists have appeared in court to explain their findings and render expert testimony.

In many instances, necropsy findings help avoid lengthy criminal investigations by first determining the species of attacker (human versus animal and, if animal, what kind). In one case, several cats were found mutilated in an urban community.[20] Concerned residents and local veterinarians feared a deranged individual was inflicting the wounds and killing the cats. Several of the cats were submitted for necropsy to the ADDL. Although significantly maimed, the cats bore the classical patterns of depredation by a coyote. A USDA Wildlife Services specialist confirmed the presence of coyote marks and scat in the areas where the cats had been found. In this case, and others like it, the ADDL was able to calm public fears and thwart a "witch hunt," saving law enforcement considerable time, effort, and money from an unnecessary investigation.

The County Medical Examiner (ME) and the OCV have collaborated on numerous cases. Unidentified remains often are evaluated by both the ME and the ADDL to determine species. Investigators from the ME have assisted pathologists from the ADDL with evidence collection from suspected animal abuse cases. The ME and the ADDL also have shared laboratory resources. The ME has a full toxicology laboratory, which the ADDL has used to investigate animals intoxicated with illegal drugs. The ME has used the microbiological laboratory capabilities of the ADDL for disease diagnostics. Recognizing their common goals and complementary resources, the ME and the ADDL have embarked on an ambitious project to build a joint facility to enhance the capabilities of both departments.

Q FEVER CASE STUDY

From 1998 to 2007, San Diego County had eight reported cases of Q fever in humans.[21] Q fever in ovine and caprine species is reportable to the CDFA, and human cases are reportable to the California Department of Public Health.[13,22] In August 2007, a woman was referred by her veterinarian to contact the ADDL with questions related to her husband's recent diagnosis with Q fever. The OCV contacted the PHS, which was investigating the 37-year-old man as a possible brucellosis or Q fever case. Staff from the ADDL, CDFA, CDC, and PHS jointly investigated the case.

The patient had numerous potential Q fever exposures: residing on a rural property which had been a cattle ranch, owning a herd of goats, hunting with his dogs, recent queening of an outdoor cat in contact with the goats, and working in wilderness areas and near a local fairground. Additionally, the patient reported cleaning bloody vulvar discharge from one of his goats and performing a "deep cleaning" of the goat areas without the use of any personal protective equipment. Onset of clinical signs occurred approximately 5 days after the patient cleaned the vulvar discharge and the goat areas. Staff from the ADDL went to the patient's residence to collect samples from the animals for testing. Sera from the goats tested negative for brucellosis at California Animal Health and Food Safety Laboratories but positive for Q fever at the USDA's

National Veterinary Services Laboratories. In the goats, the paired positive IgG titers had varying serologic changes, demonstrating both ongoing infection and past exposure to Q fever. The goats positive for Q fever were reported to the CDFA. The CDC also tested four dogs with a history of undiagnosed illness and the cat for Q fever; all were negative for Q fever by serology. A single brucellosis IgG titer from one of the dogs was negative. The most likely source for this particular case was the patient's exposure to his goats, either from direct contact or from the environment. This investigation highlights the complementary roles of local agencies and their state and federal counterparts.

METHICILLIN-RESISTANT *STAPHYLOCOCCUS AUREUS* CASE STUDY

Methicillin-resistant *Staphylococcus aureus* (MRSA) is a strain of *S. aureus* that has become resistant to some antibiotics, including methicillin. In humans, clinical signs range from mild to serious, and fatal cases are rare. Although the epidemiology of MRSA is well known in human medicine, it is not understood fully in animals. In general, companion animals are hypothesized to become infected from people but usually do not become long-term carriers. They do have the potential to transmit the bacteria to other animals and people, however.[23] Horses and pigs are the exception, with studies indicating commensal colonization.[24,25]

An anonymous call to the DEH reported a few MRSA cases among workers at a zoo in January 2008. The investigation of this report involved the PHS, the ADDL, the California Department of Public Health, physicians and veterinarians in private practice, and the CDC. The outbreak was associated with an ill baby elephant with MRSA-positive skin lesions. A total of 20 people reported skin lesions; five were confirmed as MRSA cases. All these individuals reported handling or caring for the baby elephant. All the other elephants were negative for MRSA colonization via trunk wash and rectal swab. A retrospective cohort study found a positive correlation between the number of days spent with the calf and the probability of developing MRSA-like skin lesions (Community-associated methicillin-resistant *Staphylococcus aureus* skin infections among an elephant calf and its caregivers at a zoo, San Diego, California, 2008; CDC unpublished data). The facility worked closely with the PHS and the OCV to develop and implement a plan to prevent and control the spread of MRSA. No further cases were reported after personal protection measures were instituted. Final recommendations for this facility included reminding health care providers to consider a diagnosis of MRSA in animal caregivers with skin infections and the need for standard infection-control measures to prevent disease transmission in animal care settings. As illustrated by this MRSA investigation, these agencies can work together to establish recommendations for disease prevention and control measures to improve public health.

LIMITATIONS FACED BY THE ANIMAL DISEASE DIAGNOSTIC LABORATORY

Providing quality and cost-effective diagnostic services through the ADDL is a continual challenge because of funding limitations, a shortage of skilled staff, and lack of equipment. Attracting skilled laboratory workers is an obstacle for many government laboratories because of lower compensation compared with private industry.[26] The cost of operating VDLs has increased dramatically with rising expenditures for items such as diagnostic reagents, salaries, and overhead. Furthermore, the requirements to document and comply appropriately with safety, waste management, and quality control measures have escalated. These expenses have made the cost of running a VDL prohibitive for many local governments.

The ADDL's small size and unique role have been obstacles to obtaining recognition and resources at both the state and national level. Resources available to more traditional veterinary and public health laboratories, with their respective animal and human focuses, have not always been available to the ADDL. The PHS views the ADDL as an integral part of San Diego County's rabies control program, and the ADDL staff have been trained in rabies diagnostics at the CDC. Additionally, the ADDL diagnoses 80% of the rabies cases in San Diego, and the county accounts for 10% of all rabies diagnostics performed in California.[17] The California Department of Public Health recognizes the ADDL rabies test results but has not provided financial, material, or political support for the rabies testing, as is done for conventional public health laboratories.

Major financial crises have affected VDLs in other counties, such as the closing of the Los Angeles County Comparative Medical and Veterinary Services Laboratory in 1995. The savings gained by the practice of preventative medicine far outweigh the cost of a full-blown disease outbreak. Both financial and political support are necessary to protect the public effectively.

FUTURE DIRECTIONS

Recognizing the importance of the One Health concept, the County of San Diego has embarked on an innovative project to meet current and future challenges in human, animal, and environmental health. In 2010, the county will complete construction of a state-of-the-art, 85,000–square foot Medical Examiner and Forensics Center that will bring together the OCV, the ADDL, the ME, the plant pathology laboratory, the entomology laboratory, the vector control laboratory, and the county's livestock depredation and wildlife threats program. This combination of the ME's forensic pathology expertise along with the animal, plant, and invertebrate pathology expertise is a novel experience for California and the nation. Much of the same equipment and technology are needed to diagnose infectious diseases and pests, permitting resource sharing in the new center. The co-location will foster new collaborations and innovative solutions for the county.

SUMMARY

Animal health and human health are linked inextricably. Sixty percent of households have companion animals, and almost 50% consider their pets members of the family.[27,28] This increasingly intimate relationship between animals and their human companions, which includes sharing of living spaces, provides ample opportunity for pathogens to cross the species barrier. Animal, human, and environmental health experts must pool resources to discover and address these emerging pathogens.

The ADDL's investigations of animal abuse and core surveillance programs for avian diseases, rabies, and vector-borne diseases serve as the basis for collaboration between ADDL and other departments in San Diego County. The success of these programs results from the interagency relationships and the partnering with the local community. The ADDL activities described in this article demonstrate the public health impact of a One Health approach between veterinary and human medicine. Enhanced surveillance activities by the ADDL improve public health through traditional programs such as rabies and psittacosis testing and also have led to early recognition, prevention, and control of emerging and zoonotic diseases. The ongoing collaboration between agencies in San Diego County provides a model for better disease detection and for protecting the health of humans and animals. The OCV and the ADDL encourage other local communities to develop these important collaborative relationships to protect and improve public health.

ACKNOWLEDGMENTS

The authors acknowledge the work of Dr. Hubert Johnstone, San Diego County Veterinarian for 28 years, the foundation on which the laboratory and this article were built, and that of Dr. Kerry Mahoney, San Diego County Veterinarian for 11 years. They thank Dr. Tracy Ellis, Dr. John Dunne, Brook Williamson, and Robert Lugo for editorial assistance.

REFERENCES

1. American Medical Association House of Delegates. Resolution: 530 (A-07) collaboration between human and veterinary medicine. Available at: www.ama-assn.org/ama1/pub/upload/mm/467/530.doc. Accessed January 15, 2008.
2. American Legal Publishing Corporation. San Diego County Ordinance Sec. 176.9 Recognition of County Veterinarian. Available at: http://www.amlegal.com/sandiego_county_ca/. Accessed July 1, 2008.
3. California Department of Finance. Financial and economic data: California county profiles. Available at: http://www.dof.ca.gov/html/fs_data/profiles/pf_home.php. Accessed May 9, 2008.
4. County of San Diego County Department of Agriculture Weights & Measures. San Diego County crop report 2006. Available at: http://www.sdcounty.ca.gov/reusable_components/images/awm/Docs/stats_cr2006.pdf. Accessed April 9, 2008.
5. Hawkins MG, Crossley BM, Osofsky A, et al. Avian influenza A virus subtype H5N2 in at. J Am Vet Med Assoc 2006;228(2):236–41.
6. United States Department of Agriculture Foreign Agricultural Service. FAS online United States FATUS commodity aggregation import search. Available at: http://www.fas.usda.gov/ustrade/USTImFatus.asp?QI=. Accessed May 2, 2008.
7. United States Fish and Wildlife Service News Release. Exotic parrots confiscated from smugglers returned to Mexico. Available at: http://www.fws.gov/news/NewsReleases/showNews.cfm?newsId=8ED7D2C7-0950-F2DB-9DB30E5A956367E5. Accessed May 2, 2008.
8. San Diego Natural History Museum. San Diego County bird atlas. Available at: http://www.sdnhm.org/research/birdatlas/index.html. Accessed April 23, 2008.
9. United States Geological Survey National Wildlife Health Center. An early detection system for highly pathogenic H5N1 avian influenza in wild migratory birds U.S. interagency strategic plan. Available at: http://www.nwhc.usgs.gov/publications/other/Final_Wild_Bird_Strategic_Plan_0322.pdf. Accessed April 23, 2008.
10. Kilpatrick AM, Chmura AA, Gibbons DW, et al. Predicting the global spread of H5N1 avian influenza. Proc Natl Acad Sci U S A 2006;103(51):19368–73.
11. Kugeler KJ, Gurfield N, Creek JG, et al. Discrimination between Francisella tularensis and Francisella-like endosymbionts when screening ticks by PCR. Appl Environ Microbiol 2005;71(11):7594–7.
12. California Department of Public Health. Pet bird bird laws and regulations. Available at: http://www.cdph.ca.gov/HealthInfo/discond/Documents/psittacosislawsregs.pdf. Accessed July 11, 2008.
13. California Department of Food and Agriculture. List of reportable conditions for animals and animal products. Sacramento (CA): California Department of Food and Agriculture, Animal Health Branch; March 2006.

14. California State Senate. California State Legislature AB 732. Available at: http://info. sen.ca.gov/pub/97-98/bill/asm/ab_0701-0750/ab_732_bill_19980721_chaptered. html. Accessed April 9, 2008.
15. National Association of State Public Health Veterinarians. Compendium of measures to control *Chlamydophila psittaci* infection among humans (psittacosis) and pet birds (avian chlamydiosis). 2008. Available at: http://www.nasphv.org/ Documents/Psittacosis.pdf. Accessed April 9, 2008.
16. California Department of Public Health. CA rabies laws and regulations. Available at: http://www.cdph.ca.gov/HealthInfo/discond/Documents/Rabies/CA%20 Rabies%20Laws%20and%20Regulations.pdf. Accessed July 11, 2008.
17. California Public Health Department. California rabies control program 1999–2000 annual rabies report. Available at: http://www.dhs.ca.gov/ps/dcdc/disb/ pdf/CA%20Rabies%20Control%20Program%201999-2000%20Annual%20Report. pdf. Accessed August 29, 2007.
18. Dunne G, Gurfield N, Golson D, et al. A unique veterinary and public health laboratory collaboration for enhanced rabies surveillance [Poster 23]. Presented at the World Rabies Day Conference Centers for Disease Control and Prevention. Atlanta, September 7, 2007.
19. Ascione FR. The abuse of animals and human interpersonal violence: making the connection. In: Ascione FR, Arkow P, editors. Child abuse, domestic violence, and animal abuse: linking the circles of compassion for prevention and intervention. West Lafayette (IN): Purdue University Press; 1999. p. 50–61.
20. Lau A. Series of attacks on cats worries residents: suspect sought in pacific beach. The San Diego Union–Tribune, November 8, 2001; B3.7.
21. County of San DiegoHealth and Human Services Agency. Reportable communicable diseases and conditions for San Diego County, by year of report, epidemiology statistics and reports page. Available at: http://www2.sdcounty.ca.gov/hhsa/ documents/ReportablesSummary_1991to2006.pdf. Accessed April 9, 2008.
22. California Department of Public Health. Reportable diseases and conditions Sacramento (CA): California Department of Public Health, Infectious Disease Branch; September 2005.
23. Leonard FC, Markey BK. Methicillin-resistant *Staphylococcus aureus* in animals: a review. Vet J 2008;175(1):27–36.
24. Weese JS, Rousseau J, Traub-Dargatz JL, et al. Community-associated methicillin-resistant *Staphylococcus aureus* in horses and humans who work with horses. J Am Vet Med Assoc 2005;226(4):580–3.
25. van Loo I, Huijsdens X, Tiemersma E, et al. Emergence of methicillin-resistant *Staphylococcus aureus* of animal origin in humans. Emerging Infect Dis 2007; 13(12):1834–9.
26. American College of Veterinary Pathologists. 2006 Salary Study. Available at: http:// www.acvp.org/news/salsurv/ACVP_2006_Salary_Survey.pdf. Accessed May 23, 2008.
27. American Pet Products Manufacturers Association. The 2007–2008 national pet owners survey. Available at: http://www.appma.org/press_industrytrends.asp. Accessed April 9, 2008.
28. American Veterinary Medical Association. A study pets as family members. U.S. pet ownership & demographics sourcebook (2007 edition). Available at: http:// www.avma.org/reference/marketstats/ownership.asp. Accessed April 28, 2008.

Index

Vet Clin Small Anim 39 (2009) 385–393
doi:10.1016/S0195-5616(09)00009-6
0195-5616/09/$ – see front matter © 2009 Elsevier Inc. All rights reserved.

vetsmall.theclinics.com

Every year brings you new clinical challenge

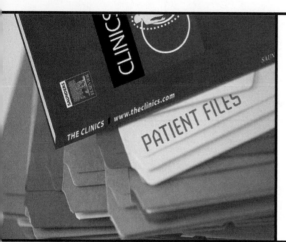

Every **Clinics** issue brings you **today's best thinking** on the challenges you fa

Whether you purchase these issues individually, or order an annual subscription (which includes searcha access to past issues online), the **Clin** offer you an efficient way to update yo know how…one issue at a time.

DISCOVER THE CLINICS IN YOUR SPECIALTY!

Veterinary Clinics of North America: Equine Practice.
Publishes three times a year.
ISSN 0749-0739.

Veterinary Clinics of North America: Exotic Animal Practice.
Publishes three times a year.
ISSN 1094-9194.

Veterinary Clinics of North America: Food Animal Practice.
Publishes three times a year.
ISSN 0749-0720.

Veterinary Clinics of North America: Small Animal Practice.
Publishes bimonthly.
ISSN 0195-5616.

M022483

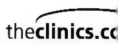